BALANCE
& other B.S.

T0386244

Felicity Harley has been a journalist for leading Australian women's publications for two decades, including a nine-year stint as founding editor of *Women's Health*. She launched and is currently editor-at-large of *whimn*. She has appeared weekly on *Sunrise* for ten years, has hosted TV shows and events and is a speaker on her favourite topics: health and wellbeing. Felicity was named one of Australia's 100 Women of Influence by Westpac for her brainchild, the 'I Support Women In Sport' campaign. She lives in Sydney with her husband, Tom, and their greatest achievements, their three children. In her, er, spare time, the health aficionado drinks coffee, does yoga, exercises (to stay sane) and cheers on the Sydney Swans. Follow her musings at: felicityharley.com or on social @felicityharley.

BALANCE

& other B.S.

How to hold it together when you're ~~having~~ doing it all

Felicity Harley

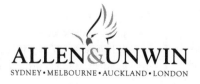

ALLEN&UNWIN
SYDNEY•MELBOURNE•AUCKLAND•LONDON

First published in 2020

Allen & Unwin
83 Alexander Street
Crows Nest NSW 2065
Australia
Phone: (61 2) 8425 0100
Email: info@allenandunwin.com
Web: www.allenandunwin.com

 A catalogue record for this book is available from the National Library of Australia

ISBN 978 1 76087 754 5

Internal design by Evi O Studio
Set in 11/17.4 pt Times Ten by Bookhouse, Sydney
Printed and bound in Australia by Griffin Press, part of Ovato

10 9 8 7 6 5 4 3 2 1

To the women in my life who inspire me daily

*Your wisdom and advice gives me comfort in knowing
we're all feeling this and the courage to pass it on*

CONTENTS

A BIT ABOUT THIS BOOK

Dear reader,

When I was mulling over how to start this book, I realised how lucky I am. I haven't had a major health crisis, I am not battling a diagnosed mental health condition, I haven't lost a child (though I did come terrifyingly close to losing one of my sons when he was just five weeks old), I haven't struggled through a divorce or experienced daily racial or other prejudice. My life has been somewhat beige in that respect . . .

But what I also am is human. I am a woman grappling with the same basic daily struggles—albeit Western ones—that you, your sister, best mate, work colleague, barista, boss, favourite podcaster or even TV host or *Bachelor* contestant or Instagram influencer are facing. No, I am not a sublime expert in feminism, but I am an expert in being a woman. I have a daughter, a mother, two sisters, one sister-in-law and four aunts, and a bunch of close girlfriends and gay friends. Whether you're single, coupled up, married, separated, divorced, a mum or not, LGBTI+ or a grandmother, I know there's some commonality in our experiences. This isn't a book to divide—I've written it to unite us. 'Overwhelm'—a handy word that I use to describe the cyclone of 1000 things going through my mind at any given time and sucking me dry—doesn't discriminate. We are all searching for more balance in our lives.

I have lived pay packet to pay packet, I've lived through an emotionally abusive and destructive relationship in my early twenties . . . not to say that these experiences increase my credentials, but I do appreciate and empathise that there are factors that contribute to our stress beyond just agonising over the twenty loads of washing you've got to do each week.

I also have a husband, Tom, who is in a demanding CEO gig (he played AFL—skippered the Geelong Cats to two premierships, in fact—and now runs the Sydney Swans). He's my feminist ally, trying alongside me to make sense of this messy time we're in, and to step up in support.

Through the adventure of day-to-day life as a woman, I am also trying to remain calm and present and be the best role model I can be for my three kids, two of whom are now in their early years at school.

For the past twenty years I have predominantly worked alongside women, editing magazines and websites that have been marketed and sold to women (*Girlfriend*, *Cleo*, *Cosmopolitan*). I spent nine years as launch editor of *Women's Health* and went on to launch women's lifestyle site *whimn*. I see the internet stories that have millions of clicks, and I write about the same topics. In many ways, my job is to know what you're feeling.

I say this with some authority because in May 2019 I wrote a piece for *whimn* that went bananas. I have never received so much feedback from friends, workmates, strangers and social media followers as I did from that article. It was called 'Balance is B.S., and modern women have been sold a lie', and it was about how we're suffocating under that mental load. I've never been asked so many times if I was okay.

I wrote that piece, and then this book, because it worries me that women's mental wellbeing is on the decline and we're sitting ducks for being sold a quick fix. There's a reason influencers are selling six-week online courses to overcome your overwhelm, 'wine mummy' memes are shared a gazillion times and companies are spruiking smelly nose sprays to stop our burnout: we are all feeling the same crunch. And it's obviously one of the reasons why you picked up this book—thank you!

One in six women in Australia will suffer depression in their lifetime, and one in three anxiety, so mental illness is common, and I want to be clear that this book is not intended as a substitute for seeking professional help. I'm writing for those of us who are quietly suffering mostly behind our closed front doors—I know we need to talk about our mental loads more, to share our stories and navigate our way through the overwhelm with our arms around each other. Like a group hug but better. We know life is good, amazing even, and we're happy most of the time, but we still need help.

In this book, you'll find there are two parts . . .

PART ONE: WE NEED TO TALK

Here, you'll find a discussion linking feminism to mental health decline, why it's happening (hello, mental load!) and, lastly, whether wellness is a true panacea to it all. It can get heavy in parts—I get ragey, exasperated and a bit pissed off. I hope you do, too. I've also loaded it with experts' opinions, studies and statistics, but stay with me as there are also ideas, thoughts and solutions in there.

PART TWO: WHEN SOMETHING HAS TO GIVE

In this bit, I aim to help you with your stress, overwhelm and your mental wellbeing, today. It's about what you can do right now to see through it all and live your version of a meaningful, healthy and well life. It's not about giving up on the feminist fight; it's about making sense of how feminism fits in today's society while still rallying on. Every chapter focuses on a 'C' word: clarity, creating space, courage, confidence and connection—so I'm running with it. Plus, it's easier for you to remember.

THE EXPERTS

I've picked the brilliant brains of some of Australia's wisest women. Feminists, social commentators, researchers, policy-makers, professors, doctors, academics—all of them living lives just like us, many also having experienced their own overwhelm. You'll love these people too. Inspiring women, including Dr Libby Weaver, Marian Baird, Jane Caro, Leah Ruppanner, Dr Ginni Mansberg, Dr Rebecca Huntley, Emma Murray, Alison Hill, Kemi Nekvapil, Lola Berry and Dana Kerford.

THE HIGH-PROFILE PEOPLE

I've peppered the book with interviews with a bunch of women I have always admired, some of whom have become friends over the years. You'll find Q&A chats with Tanya Plibersek, Fifi Box, Megan Gale, Sally Obermeder, Yumi Stynes, Kelly Cartwright and Turia Pitt. You'll like these women; they inspired me so much.

MY FRIENDS

And finally, you'll read the voices of five other women in my life. You'll see throughout the pages quotes from a bunch of my girl-friends and my two sisters. They represent a range of ages, stages, headspaces and socioeconomic backgrounds because I want you to be able to identify with someone within these pages, someone who is going through the same highs and lows you are.

Here's a quick rundown of who's who.

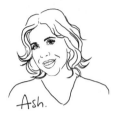

ASHLEIGH, 29

Beachside city dweller, works full-time in the media, go-getter. Oscillates between being done with Tinder and actively dating, travels, lives by the mantra 'If it's not a hell yes, it's a no'. We work together at *whimn*—a fun and bubbly desk buddy.

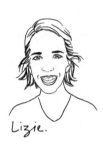

ELIZA, 34

My (not so) baby sister, lives in a country coastal town, works part-time as a marketing manager, still trying to build her career after having two girls within eighteen months. Finds solace in yoga, is a beautifully caring human. Husband is the most excellent winemaker.

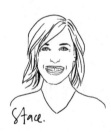

STACEY, 36

Had an uber-successful career in advertising both in London and home in Sydney. Left and studied health coaching and now runs her own business teaching mums how to cook real food. Three kids, techie husband, stylish, loves city life and quiet weekends with her family. We met at the school gate—is a burst of fresh energy when I see her each morning.

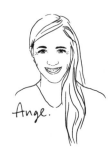

ANGELA, 40

Also a (not so) baby sister, thrives in extreme conditions, is an adventure photographer. No kids (so claims to be the 'cool aunt'), long-term partner, works mostly with blokes, rides her mountain bike for fun, literally travels the world. Her fireball approach to life is forever inspiring.

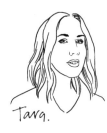

TARA, 46

Solo mum, single with two kids, from the UK. Has lived in Australia for eighteen years, works part-time as a health journalist and purposely lives away from the city. We met through work and have shared many rich conversations about life, love and wellness.

WHAT TO TAKE AWAY

When you arrive at the final chapter where I talk through all my ah-ha moments and my learnings, I hope you, too, feel inspired to speak up, are empowered to take on your overwhelm and feel clearer on this whole balance thing and the other B.S. (like wellness) that makes us feel out of whack.

Meanwhile, find a quiet space in the whirlwind of your life, grab a wine if you need, or a coffee or tea and enjoy the read. I hope my book makes you feel you are not alone, because the rest of us women are right there beside you.

Much love,
Felicity

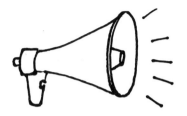

PART ONE

WE NEED TO TALK

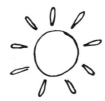

'I'm feeling strong and good and like I'm still a human being with interests and ambitions and goals I'm excited to reach.'

Amy Schumer, on returning to work three months after the birth of her son

CHAPTER ONE

HONESTLY, IS THIS WHAT WE WERE PROMISED?

All I wanted to do was go to yoga.

My husband left for work at 7.30 a.m. I finished stocking the school lunchboxes, made breakfast for three hungry stomachs, put on a load of washing, pleaded with the boys to get dressed and wrangled with my toddler over nappies, wearing shoes, blowing her nose and sucking everyone's toothbrushes. I left her with her carer, dropped my two boys at school and preschool, worked frantically for five hours and ate lunch al desko.

Around 2.30 p.m. I ducked home to collect jerseys, boots, snacks and water bottles for the boys' footy training. I grabbed the toddler first, then rushed to school pick-up and drove them all to the oval despite teary protests from the preschooler. On the way home, I felt guilty about stopping to buy takeaway noodles for dinner (no time to shop, let alone cook). Once home, I hung out that 8 a.m. load of white washing, then wrestled my yoga tights over my bum while my toddler screeched like a monkey because she was hungry.

Finally, I fed the troops.

My husband arrived at 6.45 p.m. to a home resembling a scene from *Hoarders*. I left and jumped in the car and the petrol tank

was freaking empty, so I detoured to the service station, a woman
in perpetual motion. I scored the last spot in the vinyasa flow
class, right up the front, my mat overlapping the teacher's. She shot
me a sympathetic look.

At last, I'd made it to my first yoga practice in two weeks.
I took a long, deep breath . . . then I went home and cleaned up.

Relieved? Yes! Happy? Mostly. Balanced? Hell, no.

If you buy into what society dictates as the perfect life, I have
it: married with kids, a successful career, life-enriching friends,
good health, memorable holidays and, yes, I've even got a white
picket fence. And I am grateful for each of these things (just read
my journal), even the now-grubby white fence. On the outside, it
all looks so perfectly balanced. But life is unbalanced. Messy. Off
kilter. Crazy-busy. And I am fed up.

I am overwhelmed, stressed, always 'on', tired, perpetually
guilty and burnt out. I'm always mentally shuffling my to-do
list while prepping dinner or putting away the folded clothes or
picking up footballs in the backyard, and when I am supposed to
be 'present' while listening to my six-year-old son read his nightly
school readers, I am instead back in my head, ticking off that list
again. Then I feel guilty about not being a 'mindful mum'.

In fact, this mum guilt can fast become a virus if I let those
pesky thoughts loose. Guilt around not packing healthy enough
lunchboxes, embarrassment around not making an extra effort
with Book Week costumes, shame for not whipping up those cool
macaroni necklaces from that woke mum's Instagram post. Then,
I feel even more guilty for whingeing at all when I know that women
in Syria have makeshift roofs over their heads, at best. Then there's
not replying to those 52 unread emails and . . . What about my
career—I know I'm not *leaning in* enough. What is my next step?

Hang on, those lounge cushions . . . that's right, I wanted to refresh the lounge room last year with ones I spotted at Kmart. They were so chic and cheap! Now, why didn't I do that? Oh, and also, how has my week been, health-wise? Poor. I want to get healthier. I need to drink that kale juice shot every morning, lift more weights—yeah, lift weights: that's important as my muscle mass is slowly dwindling the older I get. And what about those supplements I threw in the trolley a few months ago? I better start taking them, or that's a bucketload of money wasted (mind you, I can't start them until I've read the 21 articles I've saved in my reading list about whether they work or not). I'm also keen on running that 10-kay Colour Run with my mums' group . . . I should text them all about that to see who's up for it. And the meditation retreat I heard my yoga teacher talking about, that sounded sweet. Note to self: research places in Bali and find a friend who'll come. Actually, I'll scope it out on Instagram.

Oh boy, I need to post again to stay engaged with my social following. After I call Mum and Dad. And my sister in Canada. And my brother in France.

Arghhhhhh . . .

Yes, I even screamed out loud when I wrote that word. My life is a circus. All these swirling thoughts remind me that I NEVER have enough time for ANYTHING, especially the fun stuff: friends, exercise, meditation, yoga, reading, my career, husband, Netflix or . . . sleep.

Yep, balance is bullshit and burnout is real.

Guilt feeds the overwhelm as I try to do more, not just in my role as a mum, but for me as *me*—yes, I am still a person in all this. Aren't I?

Do we all just have to suck it up?

You might be thinking that I should suck it up and get on with life. Actually, I did a speaking gig recently in which I lamented the work–life balance conundrum and a woman, about twenty years older than me, stopped me afterwards and said, 'This is life—this is how it is. You just have to get on with it.'

To be fair, she said it kindly, but she is right—adulting, that word turned into a verb by millennials around ten years ago, is hard. So, sure, there is truth to her comment. I accept that and I often say to myself, *Toughen up. Get on with it.*

But I also feel that society and its expectations have shifted. Sometimes I feel I can't cope with all this . . . and then I run to yoga and feel better for a day. Then, the cycle starts again.

You feeling it? The overwhelm. The stress. The rage. Perhaps it's full-blown anxiety or depression.

Whether you're single, coupled up, married, divorced, a mum, LGBTI+ or a grandmother—these feelings don't discriminate. Deep down, you know you should be able have it all, do it all—perhaps not all at the same time, but you can do it nonetheless—but life is too often desperately out of control. It's the best time to be a woman, and yet instead of feeling the power, you feel so disempowered.

Actually, sometimes it's all cool bananas, you're mentally energised and you even have time to blow-dry your hair, fist pump your way to Pilates and juice your kale instead of ordering coffee on an app to save a precious two minutes. You're loving life. But then it spins out of control so quickly, so effortlessly, and you're back in the ringmaster role, hustling the circus of life around you. And so, the circle of stress begins again as you feel you need to *do* more, and *be* more to have the best life, the life which social media memes remind us of daily. And, really, all you want is a meaningful life.

Joy. Fun. Clarity. Calm.

We run countries, we run companies, we run the household and we run our kids around in the car. I am friggin' superwoman, as other women comment on my Instagram feed. Then why do I find myself picking up 938 pieces of Lego while listening to an Oprah podcast about creating more harmony in my life, throwing the cushions on the couch for the 101st time that day, hoping I will get a bolt of energy from the wellness gods to go to dinner tonight with my best friend, and wiping my son's bum while trying to read emails . . . all the while wondering, *Is this it?*

Is this what feminism is all about?

Why do I feel guilt, shame, stress and growing rage?

Because I don't know if this is what I signed up for when I stamped my feminist manifesto at age eighteen. From my many conversations with friends, colleagues, mums at the school gate and random women in the cafe and at the gym, we're *all* in this pressure cooker. We're all feeling trapped and carrying a semitrailer of mental stuff on our shoulders, but we can't find the emergency stop button. So we just get on with it.

Look, I know I've arrived at a particular point in my life when it is supposed to be busy. And, let's face it, whether you're in your twenties, thirties, forties or fifties, life today is *always* busy. If I think back to my mid-to-late twenties, boy, I was frantic with the burden of choices—career, finances, travel, mortgage and my declining fertility. In my thirties, even before I added one kid into the mix, I was juggling work with exercise and whipping up dinner at 8 p.m. when I finally made it home from the office. Now, in my forties with three children, I am always, always, always juggling and exhausted doing all of the above, plus more.

I don't just feel *too busy* though. I feel like it's all too much and—more importantly—that I shouldn't be saying it out loud. I am afraid of upsetting my feminist sisterhood and the pioneers who we owe so much. I should be able to handle it all, superwoman-style.

> ✍ 'Overwhelm for me is a hugely internalised experience, a sense that my mind can't actually take on any more information, any more requests, any more tasks or any more "Mum, Mum, Mum, Mum". I feel mentally maxed-out and physically drained which usually results in me unravelling and then resetting.'—*Lizie*

> ✍ 'An overwhelming to-do list, a feeling of foggy chaos and never enough time to fit everything in my day.'—*Ange*

A super-quick history lesson on feminism

Okay, perhaps I need to rewind a little bit, to see what exactly feminism did promise. Maybe this will put our overwhelm into context; help us understand how we arrived in this messy head-space and what's compounding it in today's world.

Let's start with the birth of feminism.

The helpful online Merriam-Webster dictionary defines feminism as 'the theory of the political, economic, and social equality of the sexes'. Social equality, I like that.

The first wave was the suffragettes fighting for political equality for women, albeit white women, in the late nineteenth and early twentieth centuries.

Then there's the modern feminist movement—the second wave—which I've always credited one woman for sparking. In 1963, journalist and activist Betty Friedan wrote *The Feminist Mystique*, which challenged the notion of the 1950s happy American house-wife. Her take: women were suppressed, unsatisfied and frustrated. While hanging out their whiter-than-white washing on their clothes lines, women the (Western) world over were shouting over the fence to each other: 'Is this all there bloody is to life?'

You can just picture it, can't you? Glamorous women with perfectly hot-rolled hair and pretty floral dresses with matching embroidered aprons slaving over their housework. And a seething dissatisfaction bubbling beneath the surface.

Thank the lord for feminism, I say. I do not want that life (apologies to my late grandmothers for any offence taken).

Friedan was often referred to as an 'accidental feminist', because she didn't realise the ginormity of the angst brewing until she started researching all this—first, for her academic mates, then for an article and, finally, for her book. She was overwhelmed by the epidemic of gloominess emanating from suburban kitchens. She labelled it 'the problem that has no name'—women drained of their individualism. Ten years later, she wrote that, like other women, she 'thought there was something wrong with me because I didn't have an orgasm waxing the kitchen floor.' If only!

The impassioned rallying cry to level the playing field between the sexes—and for women to find personal fulfilment outside the home—struck a deafening chord.

Friedan's book raised women's consciousness, alongside other prominent voices like Gloria Steinem and Jane Fonda. Australia's famous feminist, Germaine Greer, penned *The Female Eunuch*, a much-needed fire-starter in the debate.

Friedan's *The Feminist Mystique* was an instant bestseller, or, as I call it, a best-saviour. It sold a mind-blowing three million copies in three years. Nice one, Betty! And as American futurist Alvin Toffler said, it 'pulled the trigger on history'. *Boom*. This groundswell movement, coupled with advances in technology—you know, fridges, washing machines and the like—and, more importantly, the pill, released women from their 24/7 domestic drudgery (and I bet we had more orgasms) and propelled them into the workforce. Halle-flippin'-lujah.

By the late seventies, Friedan was not happy, Jan! Mind you, many were none too pleased with her either, proving it was a messy, muddy and complex feminist space. Friedan felt her movement had been hijacked by hardcore feminists, who despised families and hated men. Sheila Cronin, the leader of the feminist organisation National Organization for Women (NOW) proclaimed: 'Since marriage constitutes slavery for women, it is clear that the Women's Movement must concentrate on attacking this institution. Freedom for women cannot be won without the abolition of marriage.'

Brigid Schulte, an award-winning journalist for *The Washington Post,* puts it this way in her 2014 book, *Overwhelmed:*

> Friedan was concerned that its [the Women's Movement] attention was being diverted by 'the emotion-ridden issues of sexual politics' and 'abortion hysteria' and risked not only alienating women but failing to do the harder work of transforming the institutions and attitudes of society so that all people could do good work, sharing in raising families, and have time for life. Friedan watched mothers trying to do it all, too exhausted to be angry. She spoke to fathers who longed to be more involved with their kids, who felt so tied to work that they didn't dare try. She saw how isolated and guilty everyone felt.

Enter Friedan's new book, *The Second Stage,* which argued that families were under attack and that this needed to be the next feminism fight—for women *and men*. Worryingly, no one seemed to care.

This was in 1981, people—nearly 40 years ago—and yet I'm hearing similar cries from women and men today, about the guilt, the isolation, the exhaustion. We're all too bloody unbalanced. Sure, there has been a shift in things like flexible working arrangements, paternity leave and outsourcing help around the home, but the core of the problem still exists: women keep trying to do it all at the expense of their mental and emotional wellbeing. Empowered by feminist ideals, yet disempowered by the chance to 'have it all'.

What does a feminist look like?

You might be thinking, again, that I am a tad ungrateful for the freedom the first three waves of feminism have granted us. On the contrary, I proudly fly the feminist flag. Millennial pink, of course. I most likely fit feminist commentator Clementine Ford's label of 'nicely nicely, softly softly' feminism, which is what she called Emma Watson's HeForShe initiative in an interview in *The Guardian* in 2016. I buy into that 'soft' modern-day marketing version of a feminist and I am okay with that. Ford is far more separatist in the gender bias debate than I will ever be, but I kind of love her for that. We need loud voices, strong opinions—and ferocious rage—to mobilise the masses (that's me) to truly effect change.

I've always strongly identified with the UK's 'fun' feminist, Caitlin Moran. Her description of feminism in her excellent book *How To Be A Woman* (2011) is one you might like, too:

> The purpose of feminism isn't to make a particular *type* of
> woman. The idea that there are inherently wrong and inherently

right 'types' of women is what's screwed feminism for so long—
this belief that 'we' wouldn't accept slaggy birds, dim birds, birds
that bitch, birds that hire cleaners, birds that stay at home with
their kids, birds that have pink Mini Metros with 'Powered By
Fairy Dust' bumper stickers, birds in burkas, or birds that like to
pretend, in their heads, that they're married to Zach Braff from
Scrubs, and that you sometimes have sex in an ambulance while
the rest of the cast watch and, latterly, clap. You know what?
Feminism will have all of you.

What is feminism? Simply the belief that women should be
as free as men, however nuts, dim, deluded, badly dressed, fat,
receding, lazy and snug they might be.

Are you a feminist? Hahaha. Of course you are.

Of course, the most important thing feminism gifted us was
choice. Today, many argue that women are the most equal we've
ever been in the workplace and home (by perception, of course,
rather than reality). Sure, the gender pay gap is still at 14 per cent
in Australia, according to the government's Workplace Gender
Equality Agency. And, yes, according to the US National Bureau
of Economic Research, it is having children that creates this gap
for women in the long term, once variables such as skills and so
on have been accounted for. There are many other gaps that exist
across work (just look at the divide in industries from STEM to
tourism to hospitality) to the home front (housework, childcare),
and, of course, mental health and wellbeing.

To get a clearer picture of where feminism sits today, I decide
to talk to social commentator and author Jane Caro. I've been on
TV with Jane, discussing the news of the day, so I'm well aware
she is strong of opinion. I figure she has a solid grasp on it all,
having lived through the monumental rise of feminism in the

seventies and eighties, alongside having two kids and now young grandkids. Her 2019 book, *Accidental Feminists*, is topical.

It's a fresh spring morning when I pull up outside Jane Caro's Sydney home, in a street lined with pretty pink blossom trees. Armed with two coffees, I hear the ten o'clock pips of the ABC news as I knock on her glass front door. Her home is warm and inviting, as is her husband, Ralph, and we sit at her dining room table surrounded by vibrant art and an impressive wall of books. Ralph leaves to carry on with his work.

What I want to know from Jane is where she thinks we've gone skewiff. Where has the balance gone? Was it ever there?

'With feminism we traded flexibility because we had to do everything—when we wanted to go to the workplace for the first time, because we were now educated, the men said, "Sure, do that, but make sure my dinner is still on the table at six o'clock." What that meant was that men weren't going to change at all. Women can go into the workforce, but they still have to do all the caring of children, domestic work and mental load. Men never thought about being balanced. We were told "Women can have it all." But by "all", what *we* meant was meaningful, interesting, moderately well-paid work and a family.' Jane sighs. 'For men, that's a point of entry—they just expect that in their life. For women, it was greedy and selfish . . . it's quite bizarre how we look at the two genders.'

She nails it, doesn't she? I'm grateful I can pick her brain to help distil what's gone on before us—it's so complex, this whole damn thing. (Don't worry, she'll pop back up later to tell us more.)

To me, it's incredibly worrying how gender bias still seeps into our everyday lives in subtle (and not-so-subtle) ways. It's been wearing women down forever. Time to start speaking up.

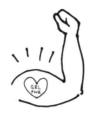

'You are responsible for your feelings and your behaviour. Draw the boundary and say, "I can't control that." Know who you are . . .'

Jane Caro, social commentator and author

CHAPTER TWO

THE PARADOX OF HAVING IT ALL, BUT STILL WANTING MORE

In my twenties, 'having it all' was a glamorised dream that had been sold to me through the media, girl power slogans and Portmans power suits. By my thirties, it grew to mean that I'd balance a successful media career with a blissed-out marriage, well-adjusted kids, perhaps Pilates, a clean house and weekends away with the girls. My first real foray into this 'having-it-all' business, however, was more smashed lollies than pretty pink fairy floss.

Let me explain. About six months into my pregnancy with my first son, I started feeling weirdly uneasy. A bit of fear mixed with uncertainty, and some excitement thrown in. The worry about work crept in quite quickly after that: concern over a loss of identity, about losing work relationships, processes, about my replacement . . . and where would 'I', my balance, fit in? I hadn't anticipated all this emotion. I thought I'd click my heels down the *Women's Health* corridors, saying, 'See ya next year!' Er, no.

I now say to my pregnant staff that this is one of the most vulnerable times in a woman's career—you're not in control anymore, you're at the mercy of those above you. You see, I went into overdrive wanting to prove I was irreplaceable . . . and then a baby came. Returning to work with my idealised view of 'having it all' was more 'having an out-of-control mess'. I was anxious and guilty about my beautiful bundle of baby fat at home, and my confidence had been somewhat smashed at work. I worried about the judgement, the gossip, especially from my staff who didn't have kids. The things I'd always prided myself on—hard work, dedication, stepping up—were now, pfft, gone. I raced out the door at 5 p.m. to start my second shift. Life was trickier, different—still good—but so different.

Now I also realise I underestimated the value of the handy skills I picked up while on mat leave: resilience, speediness, a steely focus on the task at hand and a confidence in who I was as a person as opposed to my self-esteem being wrapped up in my job title. But . . . I was busy! Having it all meant I was frantically, utterly and ridiculously busy.

Now in my forties, to me 'having it all' means doing it all and I'm done with that concept, too.

What does 'having it all' actually mean?

Let's pick apart the concept of having it all. Part of me thinks it's an outdated term, but the concept is still relevant.

I came across this quote from Michelle Obama, addressing an audience on her *Becoming* book tour in 2018: 'Marriage still ain't equal, y'all. It ain't equal. I tell women that whole "you can have it all"—mmm, nope. Not at the same time. That's a lie. It's not always enough to lean in, because that shit doesn't work.'

It's a relief to hear this from a woman whose wisdom many of us rate so highly.

But what effect is it having on our overwhelm, our stress levels and ultimately our wellbeing? Is it contributing to our lack of balance?

From my many conversations with the women in my life, I think we still get hung up on this elusive, made-up, B.S. term in our heads, at least. We might not refer to it as 'having it all', but we still have our lists, our goals, our must-dos—things we want to achieve by a certain age, etc. I mean, we damn well know that we can't have it all ... certainly not at the same time. Or ... maybe we can. So we try. But then something else falls apart—a marriage, a friendship, a job or the playdough mountain you just built. And ... then what?

Don't worry, we're reassured online. An hour of yoga will calm your racing brain.

Think about it: what does 'having it all' *actually* mean to you? Is it an outdated concept? Bullshit? Attainable? A personal goal?

Helen Gurley Brown, legendary editor of *Cosmopolitan* magazine, wrote her book, *Having It All: Love, success, sex, money ... even if you're starting with nothing,* in 1982. If nothing else, Gurley Brown popularised the idea of having it all, which was meant to be empowering. It was Zeitgeisty for a while, but somewhere along the line it's become an unattainable dream. What we're left with probably depends on how we define what it means to each of us in our own lives.

This term exists in that little brain of yours—somewhere— reminding you at age 25, 30, 35, 40, if you are not married, haven't had kids, been a boss and bought a house, then you are a failure.

You're not, but you'll feel like you are. Luckily, I knew just the woman to speak to about all this.

It's as hot as an oven inside my black car when I call Leah Ruppanner on a Monday afternoon. She's an Associate Professor of Sociology and Co-Director of The Policy Lab at the University of Melbourne. I want to chat to this expert in family policy and gender because she has conducted a bunch of fascinating studies into the socialisation of women. She might just have some answers to why we're so fatigued and fed up.

I have to call Leah from the relative quiet of my family SUV as the kids are at home, and I don't want anyone screaming at me to wipe their bum while I'm chatting to a revered expert. When I call her, she apologises for sorting her laundry into blacks and whites while she is talking to me. Suddenly, I feel . . . human. She has an American accent, and it's surprisingly soothing and understanding. As I catch a glimpse of the three car seats sandwiched in the back (don't you hate how three never fit?), I ask Leah how the hell have we arrived at this feminist state of thinking that, we, as superhuman superwomen, can do anything and everything?

'We were sold the idea that the world is equal, so you just need to step in, get your education and work your hardest and you can do it all,' Leah tells me, as sweat drips down my back. 'Then you step in and all these doors keep closing in your face. What? I can't have it all? I've been told that if I drink green juice and I meditate, then I can have it all. And if I am more mindful, and take my vitamins, then I can have it all. And I'm doing that and I feel really overwhelmed.'

Funny that. At least it's not just me. I get the vibe that Leah might be in our sinking boat, too. She has a lot of handy information that I'll share soon, but first some context.

It many ways, wanting more is just part of being human. One genius I stumbled on when I worked at *Cosmopolitan* magazine, American psychologist Barry Schwartz, has a good explanation for our angst. A smart bloke, that one. He wrote a book called *The Paradox of Choice: Why more is less* (2004). You may have heard of it before. Actually, he's also done an awesome TED Talk but, as you don't need another thing slapped on your to-do list, let me give you a quick snapshot.

Schwartz reckons choice can become overwhelming. Ummm, bingo. When you're served up too many options, rather than it being (hell-yeah) liberating, it can be (hell-no) paralysing. You are often left feeling anxious, stressed and less satisfied than if you'd had fewer options. 'More choices may not always mean more control. There comes a point at which opportunities become so numerous that we feel overwhelmed. Instead of feeling in control, we feel unable to cope,' Schwartz writes.

And let's not forget we are making choices not just for ourselves, but for our staff, our partners, kids, ageing parents . . . and the list goes on. Interestingly, Schwartz also highlights that women are nearly always the ones responsible for not only their own health—and mental health—but also the health of those around them. The other toxic element of this paradox is that good old grass-is-greener cliché—the belief that something else out there is better than what you've got. And today, if you're looking for a quick fix for this overwhelm, then there's a plethora of beguiling options, all vying for what's left of your attention.

Enter the wellness industry. I'm talking about the softer stuff: mental energy, self-care time, face masks and hot baths. This will make us emotionally balanced, won't it? Mentally strong, no?

This feeds into another paradox: female happiness. American economists and power couple Betsey Stevenson and Justin Wolfers coined this one. They researched and analysed the happiness trends of Americans between 1970 and 2005 and found that 'women's happiness has declined both absolutely and relative to men'. In the seventies, women rated their subjective wellbeing higher than men rated theirs. By the 1990s, it had switched. Let's remember here, as Jane Caro reminded me, that in the seventies women had much lower expectations of their lives and they probably said they were 'happy' because they had to be. 'Happiness is the management of expectations,' warned Jane.

But still . . . there is definitely something in this, especially if you look at the mental health stats.

> 'My life has been very back to front in regards to "the script". I had two children in my forties and my career peaked in my late twenties/early thirties. I've learned with age that literally nobody has ALL of the things (health, love, friendships, career) going for them at once and if a couple are turned up then the other things will be on simmer. I also know the story is never finished—life is cyclical and will always surprise you.'—*Tara*

Empowered, yet disempowered

I promise I am not going to bore you with an ongoing (millennial pink) feminist rant. Let's remember what Betty Friedan first wrote about: women were miserable in the home and could find greater fulfilment outside the home. True. Feminism was about giving us a sense of our own agency and ultimately boosting our wellbeing. More happiness, pleasure and joy. A sense of meaning. A belief that we could do whatever men do, whatever we wanted to do, and more. Tick, that is all covered off. But now we have a new problem looming where many of us are feeling disempowered; we lack joy, we're unhappy and we're burnt out.

As women collectively rise, our wellbeing simultaneously declines.

I'm calling it a new gender gap: wellbeing. Yet another divide between the two sexes but, unlike, say, that pesky 14 per cent pay gap, this one is growing bigger—fast.

Actually, I nicked this idea. Nah, let's say I was *inspired* by Arianna Huffington, who calls it the third women's revolution we need to have. You know her? She started the once insanely popular *Huffington Post,* had an epic mental breakdown over it, wrote *Thrive,* an exceptional book, in 2014, and then established Thrive Global with the mission of providing solutions to end the stress and burnout epidemic in workplaces. Can you tell I fangirl her?

In a poignant post titled 'The Third Women's Revolution', Huffington wrote:

Women are paying an even higher price than men for their participation in a work culture fuelled by stress, sleep deprivation, and burnout. That is one reason why so many talented women, with impressive degrees working in high-powered jobs, end up abandoning their careers when they can afford to. What we need are workplace cultures that don't make women choose between success and the wellbeing of themselves or their families. As the science shows, this is a false choice—when we prioritise our wellbeing, we're actually better and more productive at work.

This wellbeing gap starts at a very young age. I came across a worrying 2018 report called *Growing Up Unequal: How sex and gender impact young women's health and wellbeing* from Women's Health Victoria, part of the Australian Institute of Family Studies, which looked at girls and boys aged ten to twenty years old. It concluded that the 'health and wellbeing of young women was, in most cases, driven by unequal gender norms, structures and practices at both conscious or unconscious levels', influenced by parents, teachers, the media and other adults. And then these girls grow up, and like you and me, these unequal gender roles still impact our wellbeing.

I don't want to lose sight of the fact that millions of women around Australia are facing far more difficult situations than this gender gap in wellbeing. Whether it's beliefs, culture or economic factors, all women will have varying factors impacting their health and wellbeing. There are single mothers, others living in poverty, some unemployed, women shameful of the bruises inflicted by their husbands, others who have no access to affordable childcare and others still with little or no education.

As Anne-Marie Slaughter (a leading voice in the discussion on work–life balance and on women's changing role in the work-place) eloquently wrote in *The Atlantic*: 'Many of these women are worrying not about having it all, but rather about holding on to what they do have.' Her article, 'Why Women Still Can't Have It All', went bananas in 2012 as she put up her hand as a willing participant in perpetuating gen X and Y's overwhelm:

> I'd been the one telling young women at my lectures that you can have it all and do it all, regardless of what field you are in. Which means I'd been part, albeit unwittingly, of making millions of women feel that they are to blame if they cannot manage to rise up the ladder as fast as men and also have a family and an active

home life (and be thin and beautiful to boot). But almost all assumed and accepted that they would have to make compromises that the men in their lives were far less likely to have to make.

I still strongly believe that women can 'have it all' (and that men can too). I believe that we can 'have it all at the same time'. But not today, not with the way America's economy and society are currently structured.

And Australia's, too.

If you ever find the time, it's worth reading this piece in full—at the time, it was the most read article in the history of the magazine. Eight years later, every word of it still rings true.

Jane Caro agrees. 'Absolutely, mental health is a feminist issue. It comes down to women wanting to control everything and if their children are unhappy, it's their fault and if their husbands are unhappy, it's their fault. That's not true. You are responsible for your feelings and your behaviour. Draw the boundary and say, "I can't control that." Know who you are . . .'

I hear you, Jane, but it's so hard to put that into practice when you're absolutely mentally and physically depleted.

> 'I can't run my business the way it deserves and also be a hands-on mum. I have to choose and I want both. My husband gets both, but because he does, I don't. It's something I do understand, it just hurts my heart.'—*Stace*

The state of our mental health

After seeing studies popping into my inbox at *Women's Health* for nearly a decade, researching this book and most importantly talking to many women like you, I get an overall sense that our feelings of overwhelm, stress, anxiety and sheer hopelessness are rising. Swiftly.

Let's nerd out on statistics for a bit (and I promise it won't get boring). I want to give you the facts that fundamentally prove that our collective wellbeing is a bit like Donald Trump's orange tan. Yep, pretty shitty. More importantly, to reassure you that we're *all* feeling this, sister. We're all in this overwhelmed, stress-filled mothership together (kids on board or not) and, yes, life is good and we smile and enjoy it, but that fed-up feeling is forever hovering like a partner's smelly farts and it can quickly turn into crankiness, anger and rage. My friends, we will find a way out. Together.

The World Health Organization (WHO) defines mental health as 'a state of wellbeing in which every individual realises his or her own potential, can cope with the normal stresses of life, can work productively and fruitfully, and is able to make a contribution to her or his community.'

Let's look at the more serious facts first. The Australian Institute of Health and Welfare says nearly one in two females have experienced a mental health problem. And, in the past twelve months, just under a quarter of us aged 16 to 85 experienced *symptoms* of a mental health disorder. I don't know about you, but when I first read that I was like, woah, mamma! That's one in four women. Sorry, but that's a shedload. A worry, really. We're talking clinically diagnosed, more common mental health conditions like depression, anxiety and substance abuse, through to severe illnesses like schizophrenia, bipolar and personality and eating disorders.

The Black Dog Institute says 'mood disorders continue to be more common amongst women than men', particularly women aged 25–34 years, more so than any other age group. WHO agrees that gender is a: 'critical determinant of mental health and mental illness . . . gender determines the differential power and control men and women have over the socioeconomic determinants of their mental health and lives, their social position, status and treatment in society and their susceptibility and exposure to specific mental health risks.' And this is particularly true, says WHO, when it comes to rates of common mental disorders, such as anxiety and depression, where 'women predominate'.

Not surprising then that a gender gap exists in anxiety and depression rates in Australia. According to Beyond Blue, 'more women (14.5 per cent) than men (11.3 per cent) experience high or very high levels of psychological distress'. One in seven women reported suffering anxiety and one in ten depression in 2017–18. The two often go hand in hand. Other studies do confirm that men tend to be closed books when it comes to reporting mental health issues (men are at greater risk of suicide), but nonetheless the stats for women prove we need to make mental health a priority. New mothers are particularly vulnerable. Black Dog also reports that the 2010 Australian National Infant Feeding Survey showed that one in five mothers of children aged 24 months or less had been diagnosed with depression (studies since have focused on factors like C-section deliveries and mother's age at birth and its contribution to post-natal depression).

Now, what about the rest who perhaps don't fit the clinical diagnosis of anxiety and depression? The ones who can come up for happiness air, manage to exercise here and there and can laugh and still enjoy life, but then freefall into that cloudy, black mood? Well, one of the biggest national health studies conducted by not-for-profit organisation Jean Hailes for Women's Health is a clincher for me. The results of the Women's Health Survey

2018, which asked 15,262 women aged eighteen and over across Australia about all things health and wellbeing, had me nodding like a pollie in question time. Me! Yes, me! And me, too. Really, this was the deepest insight into the state of our collective well-being I had ever come across. (By the way, you can download the results of the Women's Health Survey from jeanhailes.org.au. The 52-page report contains a wealth of information, including the different ways women's responses were measured.)

Let me share the results I found most interesting:

- WE WORRY: 67% felt nervous, anxious or on edge (with 53% not able to control that worry)

- WE CAN'T SLEEP: 78% had difficulty falling or staying asleep at least several times during four weeks

- THERE'S NO TIME FOR US: 34% had no time to themselves each week

- OUR HEADS ARE FOGGY: 68% had mind blanks or struggled to concentrate

- WE STRUGGLE TO SWITCH OFF: 73% couldn't relax

- WE'RE CRANKY AF: 80% were easily irritated

Those numbers make me feel slightly better about my random mind blanks, sleeplessness and worrying . . . Like the other night when I forgot to take my contact lenses out when I went to sleep—I do this every night before I wash my face, wee and crawl into bed. So, how come on this random Tuesday night I forgot to take those slimy suckers out and woke up Wednesday with gluggy red eyes? I mean, explain that. I also accidentally missed putting my son's lunchbox in his schoolbag a few months back. I called it 'accidentally' but now I realise I simply forgot. I missed my dad's birthday last year. True story. I talked about it the night before, reminding the kids at bedtime we had to FaceTime him first thing. Then, at 8 p.m. the next day, my mum messaged me and kindly said, 'Remember it's Dad's birthday today.' Talk about, well, brain fart. I pride myself on posting the first birthday message on my family's WhatsApp group. I often forget the names of kids or friends' new partners or the cute barista or the work colleague I haven't seen for a while . . . and then wonder if I am getting early onset dementia (my grandmother had dementia in later life). Or memory loss. Or if I'm simply losing my mind. And then I worry. And think I need to do more Sudoku. Actually, I hate Sudoku.

Somehow knowing I'm not simply losing my mind makes it easier to think more rationally about the biggest pressures in my life right now; the things that overpower my sense of wellbeing. It's worth thinking about the stuff that leaves you disempowered. Maybe it's lack of sleep, a destructive relationship, finances, career aspirations, life choices, the mental load, a lack of physical activity, an incessant focus on your body, sickness within your family . . . whatever the factors, we're all experiencing this feeling of disempowerment.

I email Dr Rachel Mudge, Head of Research Partnerships and Philanthropy at Jean Hailes for Women's Health. She was the chief investigator of the Women's Health Survey. I am keen to dig a bit deeper about the findings.

'Our survey findings echo what women across Australia are feeling, namely that they're facing unprecedented pressures as they juggle work, young children as well as ageing parents and other societal demands,' Dr Rachel explains.

In her opinion, what are the main reasons why women are so overwhelmed?

'Rates of anxiety and women's negative perception of their bodies are a common theme in our survey—there's constant pressure on women to be "perfect" and effortlessly handle it all,' she writes. 'We know that the perfect life doesn't exist but when we're bombarded with images of airbrushed women on social media it's difficult to avoid feeling we're not quite achieving all we could. Being busy is also a status symbol now, so it's very easy to fall into the trap of overscheduling our lives to attain a sense of achievement.'

The survey results, of course, show how challenging and complex it is to be a woman today—the juggle of our busy lives with work, family demands, home and the increasing pressures of the digital world. Not to mention finding time for our own health and wellbeing.

'One of the biggest issues for women to improve their health is finding the time to get to a medical appointment, particularly for health checks,' Dr Rachel says.

Oh, the irony.

> 'I feel balance is a struggle I am never going to win, because honestly, I don't know any modern-day mumma who has achieved it. It's like the business world is catching up that women are rock stars—but it's our husbands and families that haven't quite caught up. They expect us to be at home and on call for them, like our mothers were, but where's the time to

work, grow our careers, to get fulfilled on that part? Heck, our mortgages are five times what theirs were, we literally HAVE TO WORK!'—*Stace*

🡕 'The biggest pressure that overpowers my sense of wellbeing is having a lack of time each day for work, play, friends, partner, fitness *and* relaxation—all of which I enjoy.'—*Ange*

Our wellbeing is stuffed

Look, I don't want to lose sight through all of this that life is good. Happy. Sweet. And, yes, there are many, many moments when we feel #blessed and #grateful, as my husband has been constantly reminding me while I've been writing this. That is very true. I don't want to whinge; I just want to highlight the strain we're all under, a strain that is tightening. (Yes, I acknowledge they are First World problems.)

We are in the midst of a wellbeing crisis. While many are suffering mental health issues, others are suffering from a wellbeing breakdown. And our physical health is also suffering. There's an enormous emotional cost—that's what I'm talking about. I want to focus on the toll gender role gymnastics is taking on our mental and emotional health. I want to focus on *you*. Yes, what *you* can do—today—in your life to clear that mental clutter, reclaim your own sense of power and, as Arianna said, prioritise your wellbeing. You know, hitting that sweet spot in your mind on a more regular basis.

This whole wellbeing-of-women concept has been kicking around since the eighties, but, for me, it's ramped up into a movement in the past five or so years. Women are craving, wanting, needing and calling out for mental space, for an increased sense of wellbeing. We're over the overwhelm. It's making us angry; the angst is building; the rage is overflowing.

How did we not see this overwhelm coming? How did we get here? What have we already lost in terms of our quality of life to the overwhelm? It is the same around the Western world—we are all feeling this. Manifested misery. This RAGE.

Okay, let's take a long, deep yoga breath.

A few years ago, before kids—when I could actually read uninterrupted—I read a book while on a work trip in the Whitsundays. It was *The Female Brain* (2006), by American neuro-psychiatrist Louann Brizendine. (Interestingly, she later came out to say male and female brains are more similar than she first thought.) There is a poignant quote in it which I have never forgotten.

> Almost every woman I have seen in my office, when asked what would be her top three wishes if her fairy godmother could wave her magic wand and grant them, says 'Joy in my life, a fulfilling relationship, and less stress with more personal time'. Our modern life—the double shift of career and primary responsibility for the household and family—has made these goals particularly hard to achieve. We are stressed out by this arrangement, and our leading cause of depression and anxiety is stress . . .

I don't know about you, but thinking about all this makes me even more friggin' tired. But I know we have to change something, otherwise this could go on and on. We're a generation of exhausted women and I want better for those who come after us, including my daughter and future daughters-in-law—and we also need to empower our partners and sons.

I'm with Anne-Marie Slaughter: I can feel the feminist beliefs on which I have built my entire career—my life, even—shifting under my feet. Could it be that a slight change of words to 'having *your* all' would allow us to take the pressure off ourselves a bit? Perhaps.

What would having *your* all look like right now? Try to set aside all your envy of other women's seemingly perfect lives. Next, set aside the obstacles you face, just for a minute. Stop blaming your partner for everything they're not doing. Don't think about your lack of sleep, your sad bank balance, your stalled career, that extra five kilos you're lugging around, your non-existent sex life or . . . I could go on. Think about what is important to you at this point in your life: family or career or hobbies or a side hustle or saving for a house. You know, the stuff that makes your heart swell with pride and ignites inspiration. Now, how do we get more of those good feelings in our soul?

It's not an easy question, but what I know for sure is that we're all exhausted and something, anything, has to give.

'Don't get so busy making a living that you forget to make a life.'

Dolly Parton, legendary singer

CHAPTER THREE

THE I'M-TOO-BLOODY-EXHAUSTED GENERATION

When you inhale the air in the Atlas Mountains in Morocco, its crispness is beautifully intoxicating. I know it sounds weird, but you can literally taste the fresh air.

I visited this barren land after I attended the annual Men's and Women's Health global conference in 2011 in Spain. Now, those were fun times. It was before kids, when life was lived on a whim. Another editor and I spent a few sweaty days mountain biking through the dusty brown hills, eating spice-laden tagines, sleeping on thin mats in local homes and shitting in dilapidated outhouses. It was rough, yet gratifying. One day, we ditched the bikes and our local guide led us on a treacherous, thigh-burning mountain hike. About halfway up, nestled inside dusty terracotta man-made walls, was a village of about 30 houses. Our guide, Hassan, led us along the potholed road, past a pack of skinny dogs, a bunch of grubby kids chasing a ball and, finally, past a man plodding along behind his cow. Washing hanging high up out of windows was gathering dust from our tracks. After walking through a muddy front garden of sorts, we arrived at Hassan's sister's house for green tea.

She flung open the door and the warmth from her toothless smile was energising. I could smell the spices in her hair. Her three young kids smiled sheepishly, while tugging at her long colourful skirt. She gave each of us a big welcome hug and ushered us into her house, and into a small room where well-worn Turkish rugs covered the floor. The dirt peeked through where the rugs didn't quite reach the walls. There was a two-seater sofa, dirty and ripped, and a vintage TV in the corner.

We sipped our tea, smiling a lot as we had a disjointed conversation through her brother. From her deep wrinkles and mostly grey hair, I guessed she was over 40, but later found out she was in her early thirties, around the same age as me at the time. She'd attended school until she hit her teens, and then married a boy from the village. She'd never left Morocco and had only done the twelve-hour trip to Marrakesh a handful of times.

As she talked, she had this supreme joy that lit up her whole face. A real delight in her eye. I asked if she had lived a good life, so far. Yes, of course, she said; she had family and friends. Food, shelter, health, animals—that was her life. She walked us through the rest of her house, which included a tiny kitchen with a sink, camping-style cooker, fridge and small cupboard, and pointed out the bedroom where her whole family slept. She then hugged me tightly as if to say, don't judge me. My life is good. I have everything I need. I live a rich, full and meaningful life.

There was a simplicity to her life that I was insanely jealous of. A happiness, an ease in many ways.

For the days and weeks after, back in the harsh reality of *Women's Health* deadlines, cover decisions, long lines of city traffic and mundane life admin, Hassan's sister's grin would pop into my mind, reminding me of another life. A mismatched world to mine. I printed out my photo with her and her children, and sticky-taped it to the side of my desktop to remind me, when I was deep in the overwhelm, that there *was* another life . . . if I really wanted it.

Technology's got us good

My life, your life, our lives are busy, hectic, rush, rush, rush. Whether you're living in a capital city or a small country town, there are increasing expectations that we have to do more, be more and in quicker time. You can thank technology for that.

Don't get me wrong—there's lots to love about technology. But here's the thing: while I don't know how I'd live without it, part of me still craves the simplicity of life before it. It's a can't-live-with-it, can't-live-without-it tug of war.

In so many ways, tech has made our lives easier (hello internet, mobile phones and laptops) and sweeter (FaceTime and Uber Eats), yet it's also made other bits a million times tougher. That processing powerhouse sitting up top (yep, I'm talking about your brain), well, it's feeling the strain of all this. Technology has altered the way we think, feel, live and sleep. The evidence is coming in thick and fast that all those apps, the 1001 emails and the social media shizzle are disrupting our thoughts, overloading our brains and fuelling our exhaustion.

Think about how TV has changed. When I was a kid, I'd get up on Saturday mornings around 6.45 a.m., ready to tape the Top 10 songs on *Rage*. At 7 o'clock the black fuzzy screen stopped and the program started. I'd hold up my cassette recorder as close to the speaker as humanly possible, ready to tape the Pet Shop Boys, Madonna and, okay, Rick Astley, too. I was always 'Shhhing' my younger siblings who talked in the middle of *the* song. So annoying. And then at 10 p.m. the snowy screen came on again.

Now, we have Netflix, Stan, Apple TV, Disney+, free-to-air TV with catch-up functions and 24/7 screen options. Seriously, how many times have you sat there in a daze scrolling up and down the Netflix homepage thinking, *There's nothing to watch*. Yet, flick over to your saved list and it's chock-a-block. The paradox of choice in action.

Not surprisingly, the impact of technology on our brains— and the mental exhaustion it creates—is a hot area of research right now. Our brains process and spit out more information and data today than they have at any point in the history of brains. Research from the University of Southern California, published in the journal *Science*, found that a human received five times as much information in 2011 as they did in 1986. (They used a complex formula that is a too-hard-basket to explain.)

Get this though: on average, we churn out, daily, six news-papers worth of info—that's the stuff we send via email, text, Facebook, WhatsApp and so on, compared with only two and a half pages 24 years ago. My grey matter hurts just writing that.

It is true that our brains have a beautiful plasticity to them— it's called neuroplasticity—and they can bend, mould and repair based on new experiences, but all this information overload comes at a cost to our mental health and wellbeing.

> ➤ *I know this might feel like heavy reading right now, but I'm including all these stats so you can get a good handle on the frightening impact of technology on our mental wellness. Stay with me here . . .*

It's been calculated that the conscious mind can process 120 bits per second, and as Daniel J. Levitin writes in his *New York Times* bestselling *The Organized Mind: Thinking straight in the age of information overload* (2014): 'In order to understand one person speaking to us, we need to process 60 bits of information per second. With a processing limit of 120 bits per second, this means you can barely understand two people talking to you at the same time. Under most circumstances, you won't be able to understand three people talking at the same time . . .'

Just ask my kids about this.

Then, there is the subconscious mind—the stuff that happens that we're unaware of. Say, for example, when you drive home from work and you spend the entire time thinking about work, what you have to do when you get home, dinner, the weekend, your gym schedule for next week, and then you pull up outside your house and—blimey, what just happened? Do you remember any of that drive home? Nope. It always freaks me out when I have those journeys. We have so much information feeding our subconscious mind, plus all the thoughts processing in your conscious mind, and the bottom line is that 'it's clear why many of us feel overwhelmed by managing some of the most basic aspects of life,' says Levitin.

So it's not just me!

Just quickly, what's the first thing you do in the morning: check your phone? The last thing you do at night: check Instagram? Please don't beat yourself up over wanting to check social media for the 29th time today. We all do it. In fact, an American study found we check our phones every twelve minutes. Four hours is the longest stint we're prepared to keep our hands off them. And hold the phone for this: one in three Australians say they are addicted to their phones. You too?

It's really hard. I get it. Phone separation anxiety is a real thing. Actually, technology and the information it delivers is a bit like sugar: we get addicted to it. There's actual proof our brain wants to take in all this new information—subconsciously or consciously—and we also feel like we have to. To keep up, to fit in with our peers, workmates—it's part of being human. We use information to find that common thread to validate connection. The watercooler chat over the latest bloke booted out of *The Bachelorette*, why Bikram yoga has been replaced by cold-room workouts, what Meghan Markle ate for breakfast, Brexit, Syria, Russia . . . we should know all that, right?

Technology, and our constant need for information, can easily sap our time, overload our brains and magnify our stress . . . if we let it.

Wake up, say a prayer and hustle

Thanks to technology, we have given new meaning to the word 'hustle'. Think of memes like 'Wake up. Kick ass. Repeat' and 'Hustle until the haters ask if you're hiring' that intend to motivate but seem to irritate. The Instagram stories of speakers/writers/experts/entrepreneurs aka 'slashies' who are networking here and hashtagging (#grit #werk #slay) everywhere. The mums who exercise at 5 a.m., then work on their side hustle for an hour and whip up enviable school lunchboxes all before heading off to their fully paid job . . . and have a YouTube channel so we all know about it. And what about 'My Day on a Plate' columns and the perfect eating plans of people who activate their almonds. Not to mention the 'How I Get It All Done' feature articles that make you realise there's absolutely no way you'll get even half of it done. And even the hero of hard work, Beyoncé, is in on it, singing in her feminist anthem 'Formation' about dreaming it, working hard and grinding until she owns it.

Hustle, hustle, hustle, on, on, on, do it all, do it all . . . it's EXHAUSTING! All this 'living your perfect life' sales pitching is part of so-called hustle culture—our society's standard that you can only succeed by ensuring you're always running at 100 per cent. I don't remember Betty Friedan recommending we do that.

From the moment you wake up to when you go to bed, you're 'on', 24/7. Yep, always available and always reading about how other people are working and hustling more than you. You know the type—actually, you might be one of them (I have been, I am!)—obsessed with striving for productivity and perfection, particularly on the work front. That treadmill of comparison makes you feel like shit a lot of the time. It's a vicious cycle that ultimately leads to, you guessed it, burnout.

Actually, our use of language has a lot to answer for: 'I've got so much on'; 'I'm so busy'; 'I'm under the pump'. Living life on the go is cool. Superhuman, somehow; glamorous even. Often when you constantly tell people you're busy, you want people to perceive you as having higher social status (you're not going to consciously think this, of course, but that's often the underlying motivation). As a society we hate being bored and our culture of busyness—do more and do it all—and the value we place on it is the ultimate stress trap.

> *Sometimes I also wonder whether my chaos is compounded by having too much stuff (I'm sure Marie Kondo would agree). Our culture is bloated with goods, be it clothes, plastic toys, furniture, home-delivery meals, sneakers or sheet masks.*

When I was 22, my sister Ange and two friends and I did a road trip from Vancouver down to Vegas during the July break from uni. We taped a handwritten black texta sign, saying 'Vegas or Bust', to the back window of our mate's beat-up old truck. We stayed in cheap hotels, drove all night, kissed random guys and snapped hundreds of photos on our Kodak film cameras. We'd call our parents every few days while we were stopped at a gas station, using a calling card on a pay phone. Once my $2000 of savings dried up, I flew back home to the reality of my part-time waitressing job and study.

Whenever I think about all this hustling we do now, my mind zaps back to the time I rode that ridiculous roller-coaster on top of the New York-New York Hotel & Casino in Las Vegas at the end of that trip. It sits sky-high on the roof of the casino and twists and turns as it snakes over faux New York buildings. That Las Vegas roller-coaster represents life in many ways. At the time, that ride was exhilarating, and thinking about it reminds me that things were a lot simpler back then. Carefree. Idealistic. I had balance, albeit with epic hangovers. I was innocent of the trappings of modern society in many ways. Looking back, it seems that as society progresses—and as I get older—year after year, our roller-coasters are upgraded. They get more elaborate, trickier, scarier and faster.

I want to jump off the roller-coaster I'm on, but I also don't want to miss out on the thrills and laughs along the way. That's the dilemma, right? There's a great quote from the old-school movie *Parenthood*, that one starring Steve Martin and Keanu Reeves when he was about 25. It's from the grandma who had been on a roller-coaster when she was nineteen. It goes like this.

'I always wanted to go again,' she says, 'you know, it was just so interesting to me that a ride could make me so frightened, so scared, so sick, so excited and so thrilled all together. Some didn't like it. They went on the merry-go-round. That just goes around. Nothing. I like the roller-coaster. You get more out of it.'

How true.

Isn't this part of the paradox? You want it all (the roller-coaster), but there's a price to pay for those highs and lows. Would you prefer the safety of the merry-go-round? Probably not.

I want you to take a moment to think of other things that add to your daily overwhelm. The stuff that just complicates life that little bit more and multiplies the brain fog. It might sound all a bit simplistic, but seriously, that DIY Coles check-out beeping at you to call the attendant for the fifth time can stress people *out*. I've witnessed some admirable meltdowns over 500 grams of mince failing to scan. There are plenty of things that start small and escalate: bills piling up, Centrelink bureaucracy—and don't even start me on the palaver you go through if you've forgotten your Apple password . . .

I think Brigid Schulte nails it in *Overwhelmed* when she says: 'Technology spins that overwhelm faster.'

> 🖉 'I feel like a lot of hustle culture revolves around optics. We wear 'busyness' as a badge of honour and social media has only amplified this.'—*Ash*

The unchanging workplace

We believe that our devices need to be within reach at all times—after all, it's this technology that has granted us the flexible working environments that have given women so many great opportunities. But I suspect the workplace is actually adding to our overwhelm and inhibiting our wellbeing. That devices have turned workaholism into a lifestyle.

Who better to turn to with this theory than Marian Baird, Professor of Gender and Employment Relations at Sydney University? The esteemed academic is one of Australia's leading researchers in the field of women, work and care. She works with government departments, organisations, unions and not-for-profits to improve the position of women in the workforce and society. Her research was instrumental in the genius piece of legislation that gifted us paid parental leave. She's nabbed an Order of Australia, too. Cue a collective round of applause for her tireless work for all women. She truly knows the feeling of 'how on earth am I going to do this?' as she has raised four kids, juggling work, home and life.

It's Monday morning and Sydney Uni is dripping in sunshine. The students could be skipping class for all I care . . . I am revelling in the sun, baby. It makes me happy and reminds me how truly beautiful life can be. I am on my way to grab a quick coffee with Marian. She waves to me across the concourse; she reminds me a bit of my mum—warm and wise.

Marian gets straight to the point.

'The big shift that happened is that workplaces became far more intensified and expectations raised. That's the missing bit of the puzzle,' she says while slowly sipping her coffee. 'In the eighties, there was a rise of the Japanese "lean organisation" and a huge shedding of labour, so we were expected to do more tasks on the same money. The way women have responded in Australia is to work part-time. So, in 40 years, there hasn't been a single uplift in full-time work for women—all the growth is part-time. Full-time rates for women are actually slightly lower.'

I think about my twenty years as a journalist, and how in my first job at *Girlfriend* magazine I wrote about five stories a month. Five stories! That's it. Now, at *whimn*, the women fresh out of uni are writing up to five stories a *day*, plus editing, picture researching, building the story in the content management system, pressing send and then putting it out on social media. Not to mention interviewing, nurturing their PR relationships and coming up with killer ideas. Phew.

I get it, we are all proud we can 'do everything' at work and so we should be. But where are the boundaries between work and life? Where's the space for mental downtime? Reality check: there isn't any. Those boundaries? Yeah, they're flimsy AF. Whether you're a white-collar worker or making ends meet, there are no barriers anymore. You are 'on' between 6 a.m. and 10 p.m. all day, plus weekends. Even if you're only supposed to work part-time ... forget about it, you're still plugged into work on your off days. Say you take a twenty-minute call on a Saturday morning with your company's US office, but that turns into 40 minutes plus prep time and wind-down time, and there goes a precious two hours of your weekend. You know, the two hours you had planned to exercise—pfft—vanished.

Since we entered the workforce, women have internalised the mindset that to get ahead we must work harder, longer hours and always be available to our boss, team and, nowadays, to some random commenting on our social post. We have different expecta-tions of men and women in the workplace. There is increased value around workers who are available 24/7 and have no domestic load at home. Really, this is a dude clutching a briefcase from the 1950s. This always-on mentality has hit millennials and xennials (yes, me, the microgeneration in the middle of gen Xers and millennials) the hardest because our jobs have involved, yep, technology.

When I was writing about this issue for *whimn*, career management expert Sally-Anne Blanshard told me that's it down to the evolution of the workforce. Just like Marian lamented. 'Technology has changed our expectations surrounding commu-nication so we're always "wired" for work,' Sally-Anne says. 'Companies offer laptops, phones, and this by its very nature means that the expectation is to be on all the time. But does your energy match this?'

While women have entered the part-time workforce in droves, too often we end up doing a full-time gig in shorter hours. While flexibility was meant to be family-friendly (and, interestingly, women who work flexibly often feel more confident at work), it too often creates more stress. In her book *Fair Play*, Eve Rodsky, a Harvard-educated lawyer turned organisational specialist, coins a genius term—the 'she-fault' parent. She writes: 'In our culture, "mom" has been deemed as the she-fault, de facto household manager and caretaker.' Who answers the call from school when your child's fallen over and bumped his head? Who has to leave early to let the washing machine repairer in? The part-time worker. But then she is expected to answer her emails while waiting at the doctor's to see if her son's head is okay. And then finish her report on the weekend because that washing machine repairer never showed up.

This work–life conflict can grind you down, it takes up mental space—and energy—as you never really switch off.

These feelings support 'the four-day fallacy': you're paid for four days, and work five (at least).

> ➘ *Eight hours of paid employment a week (no more, no less) significantly boots mental health and life satisfaction. This little tip comes courtesy of the helpful researchers at the University of Cambridge.*

And this, my friends, is what experts say is one of the biggest contributors to women's stress. Companies know that the majority of women want to work like this—with or without kids—and, yes, they take advantage. They are savvy to the fact that women are willing to demonstrate their gratitude, and thus will work extra unpaid hours, to prove their worth. Confession: I have fallen victim to this but I have also—subconsciously—thought this about some of my part-time staff. I just know they will work harder. In September 2019, Andrea Cross, a businesswoman and the New South Wales representative of the pay equity lobby group Business and Professional Women, told the *Sydney Morning Herald*: 'It sounds like the answer to balance but it rarely turns out like that in reality. Companies use the promise of flexibility to woo women but often it turns out to be lip service. You have employers knowing that the women want these flexible hours, they are desperate to keep their job and they need the money as much as anything else, and the employers quite often can make strong demands on women's time. And women just can't afford to say no.'

All round wise woman Marian Baird believes it's actually impossible for two full-time workers with children in Australia to keep some sort of family balance. In my experience, she's right. Tom and I tried it and everyone's wellbeing, and our marriage, suffered. I often read headlines such as 'Parenthood is extraordinarily hard' and 'Mothers on the brink' about both parents working hard to make ends meet. I've wondered if it is a city problem as mortgages and living expenses are higher. But then friends who live outside the big cities remind me that it's a strain everywhere.

I also think it's easy to be blind to this unspoken workplace inequality. Before kids, I naively thought both Tom and I could still maintain our full-throttle careers and didn't truly appreciate the toll that would take on our kids, and on us individually.

Marian says, 'I am waiting for the resentment to blow up with your generation . . . I went through a period of resentment and then I got over it. It's a marathon that you're working so don't sprint at the beginning, you'll burn yourself out, collapse, especially when you've got young children. But if you do want to have a career, and most young women do, you still have to maintain a connection with the workforce.'

'Oh, don't worry,' I tell her, 'the rage is building.' I am angry. I know, collectively, we're all pretty fed up with this current arrangement. So how come my career comes second to Tom's all of a sudden, just because my earning capacity is less?

'We don't have a culture where we have someone living with us to help us,' Marian says. 'A lot of us have used a nanny a day or two a week, or someone coming to clean the house, and a lot of people don't talk about that.'

I confess to Marian that we have had the same amazing nanny for four years, Carly, who is an extension of our family. I'm often embarrassed to talk about having this part-time help, as I worry what other women will think—that life is easier with home help. Mind you, most of my wage goes to her.

Marian stops me mid-confession. She asks, 'Is it *your* wage or is it a combined wage?' Before I can answer, she says, 'We have to change our language around that. That's how deeply ingrained norms are—they are very hard to shift. A lot of people say, "things have changed but it's not got any better". It has, but things are different. There is a lot more recognition of women in the workplace, monetarily, if they have children but the structure of the workplace hasn't changed.'

From the pay gap to discrimination, being passed over for opportunities, feeling invisible and always being on—have you felt any of this? Me too. This inequality between how males are treated at work compared with women fuels our cynicism and frustration with the whole work–family balance . . . and you bet we're burnt out.

⤴ 'It often feels like someone turned the dial up on the treadmill and it's only getting faster. There is a demand to do more, be better, stay competitive, ideate quicker, remain relevant while pushing the boundaries—produce work faster and at a higher level of quality than yesterday . . . and do it in less time with less money. It's fun, exciting, challenging and has stretched me in more ways than I ever could have imagined, but it also makes you feel that if you stop to take a breathe the world might run away without you.'—*Ange*

. . . and we're burnt out

We throw the burnout word around pretty liberally, but what does it actually mean? Is it a medical thing or a social condition? Is burnout just a workplace thing?

I quite like Belgian philosopher and author Pascal Chabot's take on burnout: he calls it 'civilization's disease'. This expression sums it up delightfully as a health concern we ALL need to care about.

In May 2019, WHO officially labelled burnout as an 'occupational phenomenon' and added the word to its handbook, the *International Classification of Diseases*. Their definition of burnout is 'a syndrome conceptualised as resulting from chronic workplace stress that has not been successfully managed.' They highlighted three key things that I'm sure you can identify with: feeling utterly exhausted, not being kick-arse in your job in the ways you normally would be and mentally checking-out.

I don't know about you, but I've felt all of these outside the workplace. Were these caused by the workplace? Not necessarily— I would say it was more about the collision of stressors from work *and* home that caused me to feel, well, burnt out. Reduced. Distant. Exhausted. Over it.

Linda and Torsten Heinemann, authors of a study published in the journal *SAGE Open*, suggest that burnout has become 'one of the most widely discussed mental health problems in today's society'. I tend to agree. And I can't help thinking it's a mental health problem that hits women a hell of a lot harder than men, because of that collision again: work and the home front.

A study from Montreal University of 2026 people (half women, half men) found women suffer from alarmingly higher rates of burnout than blokes. Main reason? Women were less likely to win positions of power, which means we make fewer decisions and use our skills less, which leaves a lot of us frustrated and defeated. The study concluded that these gendered working conditions fuel lower self-esteem—as women have more difficulty balancing work and family life (no kidding)—and the female respondents also felt work encroached on their family time more than it did for their blokes.

My go-to sociologist, Leah Ruppanner, attributes some of the blame to our employers. 'Organisations need to acknowledge their workers have demands outside of work and look at how can they create a workplace that truly supports this. A lot don't. If you support them, people are happier and their productivity goes up.' Win-win.

In my experience, a company can have—and sell—a 'family-friendly' policy, but it's the direct manager who interprets the rules. Work burnout comes in many different forms and is an entirely individual experience. When I asked my friends about a time in their lives when they felt completely and utterly burnt out, every one of them could precisely recount the days, weeks and months.

⊿ 'I didn't know what burnout was until I took a four-month sabbatical and looked back on how tired I had become from constantly producing and creating. I took the time off to do a personal photo project but instead realised that my creative soul just needed nourishing and it was okay to just be.'—*Ange*

⊿ 'In my late twenties climbing up the career ladder, I was editing three magazines at once. I felt completely unable to say no to anything workwise and I got burnout in the true sense of the word. I was rushing everywhere all the time, I hated it.'—*Tara*

In need of a better way

Those Atlas Mountains are feeling so inviting right now—the tranquillity of the isolated surrounds, a slower speed of life, freeing oneself from time constraints. Less tech, too. I just pulled out some pictures from that merry trip, to remind myself of Hassan's sister's face, to see her grin, to feel her calming energy. It still makes me smile.

There's a photo of me sitting on a sharp rock, alone, with hardcore walking boots and a backpack on. I am perched at the top of the mountain gaping at the glorious view. I remember this photo being taken; I remember feeling utterly in awe of the sight of a country so different to ours. Seriously though, packing up our lives and moving to Morocco is by no means the answer to my chaos. A visit there might help, but our lives are here right now.

So, surely, there has to be a better way of doing things? Surely we can sort through this mess?

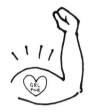

'Changing the way you work when your life changes is a normal, rational, sensible thing to do. But somehow we're stuck on the idea that it's a normal, rational, *lady* thing to do.'

Annabel Crabb, journalist and author

CHAPTER FOUR

THE SECOND SHIFT

Each night, as I was writing this book, I'd discuss my various interviews and research with Tom—usually a hurried conversation over the circus of dinnertime. Often, he would raise the point: but what about men? They are feeling this overwhelm, too. They want to be more engaged, more connected. They are torn between work and family life—they have little or no balance, either. Men aren't able to live up to the new set of husband rules that we, as *soft* feminists (remember), bring to the table when we recite our wedding vows. He is confused.

I'm a bit confused too, because, you know, I think he's right. But I still feel . . . angry. It's not like Tom sits there with his feet up watching Fox Sports after dinner—he's mucking in, cleaning up, bathing, navigating homework. Mind you, he can sit and watch TV on weekends, surrounded by chaos; his housework timelines are more forgiving than mine.

Remember, men have to want to change, and thankfully he does. I know other husbands who just clock-off when they clock-on at home—where's their incentive when they already have it pretty sweet? The simple fact is that I carry the load of the household concerns up there in my head: the planning, shopping, finances, dinners, holidays, childcare, friends' party schedules, the dentist appointments—it just somehow falls to me.

As an aware feminist husband, Tom asks to help, but dear god sometimes I wish he would just get on and do it without asking.

Men, we're talking to you

All the experts I've spoken to so far—Jane, Marian and Leah— believe that men need to be part of this conversation, too. Rather than engaging in feminist warfare with them, we need to empower men to ask for time off, to leave work earlier to do school pick-up, to be the on-call parent for day care.

'The research shows that men more than ever want to be engaged in family life in ways their fathers didn't,' says Leah. 'They want to be more connected, they don't want to work as much as they do. They want more time for their families. But what makes me a little enraged is when men shut down and say this is just another feminist ragey thing. The data is the data. They can't dismiss the whole argument as feminist nonsense, they need to recognise the facts and then step into the conversation. Men are in positions of power and are more likely to be able to change the corporate rules and institutional models that haven't moved since the 1950s.'

Marian agrees that the time is ripe for a wider discussion. 'We've got to the point now where nothing is going to change unless the men change. The women have done everything they can,' she says.

It's this very topic that ABC political writer and comment-ator Annabel Crabb tackles in her 2019 Quarterly Essay, *Men at Work: Australia's parenthood trap*. She discusses how women have adapted to the demands of the workplace—particularly after the birth of their first child—while men haven't budged. The men who want to move—for example, who ask for flexible work hours or to perhaps leave a little earlier so they can coach their daughter's footy team—are often discriminated against. Apparently this is called 'flexism', meaning the everyday and subtle discrimination targeted at flexible workers (yep, those workers attempting to find more family life balance in their days). Crabb writes:

> The average Australian father worked five hours more a week after the birth of their first child. And if we're serious about women's participation in the workplace—and given the double shift worked by the majority of working mothers in this country, that can only feasibly be achieved by giving them a hand at home—then that means being serious about men having the opportunity to leave it when they need to, just like women do. Changing the way you work when your life changes is a normal, rational, sensible thing to do. But somehow we're stuck on the idea that it's a normal, rational, *lady* thing to do.

My trusty feminist ally Jane Caro says this work–life gender disparity will continue to gain force until more men step up. In her book *Accidental Feminist*, she puts it this way:

> The day-in, day-out work of parenting and home and personal maintenance remains stubbornly intransigent despite all the whizz-bang labour-saving devices. What has changed is the expense of buying a house, paying a mortgage and running a household and a car (or two), bringing up kids and paying all the bills that go with them. As we all know, it now takes two incomes to simply keep a family's head above water, particularly in our major cities. The earner of one of those incomes, usually the woman, still shoulders the lion's share of all the other unpaid work required. She pays a high price for this not just in terms

of exhaustion, but also in terms of loss of time (and energy) to devote to her paid work. This means she often works part time, or even if she works full time gets overlooked for promotions and pay rises. It is a circular bind that some of my generation and our daughters have found themselves caught up in. The sheer weight of the unpaid work women do impacts on their ability to find higher-paying work. Their lower income then leads to both partners accepting that he should work longer hours and she should take on more of the housework, which impacts on her ability to get paid work, which . . . and round and round we go. It's a vicious cycle that gathers speed as women age, until it becomes a tornado.

A tornado! Yes. That's why I can feel a storm brewing. And this, dear readers, is also why balance does not exist and—oh, there goes our wellbeing.

> ⤴ 'For me, it was the six months after having each of my three children. It's the point where you feel like you're never going to get sleep and your business is starting to really suffer without your TLC. People stop checking in and the nights seem so much longer. Hubby is back at work kicking goals, bigger kids realise this tiny human isn't going away and they're resentful too.'—Stace

Home work

When I fell pregnant with our first son, I felt I was at my career peak—*Women's Health* was flying and I was professionally enriched. Alongside work, Tom and I travelled and hung out with friends; I did yoga, I had 30-minute baths with sheet masks,

I watched TED Talks, I cooked from books by inspiring women I fangirled, like Michelle Bridges. Tom would knock up a nice spag bol, he'd spruce up the garden. Life was nice.

It's funny how you innately fall into predictable gender-based roles. I'd taken control of cleaning inside, and it was probably more like 60/40 on the housework front, but I put that down to my clean-freak nature. Or was it because our definitions of clean are different (how could he miss those crumbs on the bench)?

It took me eighteen months to fall pregnant. It could've been my age, but I'd had appendix complications in my twenties, so I was carrying a bundle of scar tissue in there, or perhaps it was my stressed-out-about-fertility mindset. You see, when it finally happened at age 35, I'd just returned from another epic work trip to New York City (shopping, eating, drinking) and I'd come to the mindset that if I couldn't have children, I would be okay. I mean, Oprah never had them and look at her legacy. Life would roll on and I'd find enrichment elsewhere—wider family, nieces, nephews, friends, travel, living overseas again, giving back in places that had left imprints on my heart like Guatemala, Cuba and Morocco, of course. Life would be easier, somehow.

Then—tah-dah—a faint blue line appeared. Up the duff. And I was downright ecstatic. In due course, I left *Women's Health* in the trusty hands of my 2IC and went on mat leave.

And at 2.34 a.m. on a steamy February night, my life changed forever. In a Sydney hospital operating room, a sixteen-hour labour ended with an emergency caesarean and the birth of my son. My priorities shifted. And my load exponentially grew.

It's that second shift: the work you do at home before you go to work, and again when you get home and through the night. Or if you don't work, then all day and on the weekend. I'm sure our feminist foresisters hoped we'd be doing less of it all by now and freeing up our spare time, our mental space. This second shift kicks into full throttle once the first baby is born. It seems that the introduction of kids traditionalises everyone. Even more.

> ✈ *I talk about the mental and emotional load in Chapter Five. Here, I'm primarily talking about the unpaid physical work that we do that's fuelling our stress and rage.*

It's a fact: women do a shedload more work around the home. I mean, because you've got a vagina you're better at mopping the kitchen floor, right? (Don't forget it might just be followed by an orgasm.) Another thing that makes me weirdly ragier is calling it 'unpaid work'. The OECD, that's the Organisation for Economic Co-operation and Development, defines unpaid work thus: 'Work that produces goods or services but is unrenumerated. It includes domestic labour, subsistence production and the unpaid production of items for market.' Simply, if you can pay for the job to be done, it's unpaid work. Stuff like walking the dog, logging your online grocery order for the week, washing your outside garbage bins (Do you do that? Ours stink!) or driving your grandmother or mother or aunt to their heart specialist appointment. Yes, you, my friend, are the CEO of the household economy, and often the CFO too. Yeeha.

It's a cold, hard fact that women spend more time doing unpaid housework regardless of whether they are single or working full-time. According to the 2016 Australian Census, while we spend between five and fourteen hours on housework *per week*, blokes do less than five. If you're single, you will be loading that dishwasher slightly more times than a man does—that is, even

when it's just housework for one, women will spend more time
on it than a male equivalent does. When you shack up, regardless
of your or your partner's work hours or income, your housework
goes up a little, while his goes down. Then—boom!—along comes
the first baby and men's hours pretty much stay the same. The
women adapt, the men relax. The epic *Household, Income and
Labour Dynamics in Australia Survey*, aka HILDA Survey, which
followed just under 20,000 Australian households over sixteen
years, found that, yes, women do far more housework than men,
and as the children grow up, it only gets worse.

> ⍚ *Use this one next time you're nagging: when both people carry
> their load of the housework, that couple has more sex. This
> 2015 study from the Uni of Alberta involved 1300 couples, so I'm
> buying it.*

I'm forever envious of Tom for not seeing the toy explosion
in our tiny backyard or the Everest-size mountain of unfolded
washing on our lounge or the *Frozen* dolls with their pretty
heads stuck in the sandpit. He can kick back and watch sport and
somehow switch off from the chaos. Take time out for his mental
wellbeing. Why can't I do that?! And then, I'll walk around slam-
ming the plates in the dishwasher because someone left them in
the sink when HOW HARD IS IT TO PUT YOUR CEREAL
BOWL IN THE DISHWASHER? Granted, he tells me to leave
it and he'll do it later and, once again, I'm bewildered as to how
he can switch off from the chaotic mess. I huff and puff in my
pissed-off state, picking up the crap lying on the kitchen bench;
I storm down the hallway with the washing basket to put the

clothes away, and I slam down the toilet seat and say, 'Oh sorry, was that a bit loud?'

This behaviour is called 'rage cleaning'—it's when you constantly clean up after other people, when they could easily do it themselves, and you get cranky in a passive-aggressive way.

I believe another big reason we have no balance and little time for ourselves is because we, as women, can't step away from the dishes, walk past the unmade beds *again* and keep stuffing the recycling under the kitchen sink. You know, I am writing this book on the free desks at my local library because I have to keep out of the house, because of the lure of . . . you guessed it, housework!

> ♪ 'My burnout happened when I had a seventeen-month-old, a newborn and a husband working seven days a week, while moving to a new house and attempting to come to terms with the fact that my sense of self was absolutely nothing.'—*Lizie*

Mum. Mum. MUM!

I did a little experiment the other day: on average, when my preschooler son has just done a poo, he calls out 'Mum' three times before he calls out 'Dad' to wipe his bum (yes, a lot of bum wiping goes on in our house). My eldest son calls me to retrieve the footy that he's kicked onto the shed roof, and I climb up the stepladder in my pink slippers and nearly get bitten by a spider. Don't get me wrong, there is something heartwarming about this but it's also heart-worrying.

As I am writing this, I am thinking and feeling and examining my raw heart, and I don't carry any deep resentment. I'm okay as it's a choice I made. I accept that. Sure, I carry surface day-to-day resentment, exasperation and frustration. If you have kids, I'm sure you feel the same. As any mother would know, children bring a profound new love and richness into your heart. Before kids, I was naive to the *real* impact of the second shift. Naive to the emotional, mental and physical side of parenting. Naive about how it would mess with my marriage at times. Naive about how much time it all takes up. Naive about how it would ultimately affect my wellbeing.

'We shouldn't underestimate that all of this labour requires mental energy to ensure the hamster is alive and the dishes are unloaded. It is no wonder we're increasingly feeling time pressed, stressed and depressed,' says Leah.

No surprises that mothers are 18 per cent more stressed than other people. That might sound like a strange statistic to arrive at, but boffins from Manchester University and the Institute for Social and Economic Research at Essex University asked an impressively sized sample of women, 6025 to be precise, and examined eleven indicators of chronic stress, like hormones and blood pressure. They found that working mums with two kids had 40 per cent higher levels of chronic stress. Women who had flexible hours and worked from home were no less stressed. Add all of us into the mix, and we're talking a lot of stressed-out women. Pass me a bottle of wine. *Now.*

Dr Inga Lass, a research fellow of Applied Economic and Social Research at the University of Melbourne who worked on the HILDA Survey, told the *Sydney Morning Herald* at the time the study came out: 'Women have to find ways to combine housework, care work, and their paid work, whereas men can be much more focused on their employment. I think this is directly related to women feeling more stressed.' Dr Lass believes the gender wage gap is partly to blame.

Let me refer to Eve Rodsky again who, for her book *Fair Play*, wrote down every single thing she did day-to-day on a 'shit

I do' list, to quantify the time. Her list doubled and tripled as she tallied every time-sucking detail of her physical and mental load. She was left gobsmacked by the imbalance beween what she did versus what her husband did. She triumphantly emailed her list to her husband. His response: the monkey covering his eyes emoji. She then asked her friends to do the same.

Leah advised me to stop doing everything for a week. Stop doing it all. Just *stop*. I lasted one day.

One weekend in footy season when Tom was away, it was particularly rough. One kid had a cold, another would not sleep. I tried a trick that made me feel more valued in a way—I totalled up the number of hours I was 'on' between 6 a.m. and 9 p.m. and realised it came to about $2000 (pre-tax) worth of work time. For two days. I texted this to my mum friends. The emoji replies were rather hilarious and sweetly reassuring.

Weirdly, I had a dream that weekend that Tom, his mates from his footy days and I were renting an Airbnb, who knows where. They all left early and I had to do *all* the cleaning up as I was so scared my rating would be ruined. The next morning, while processing the dream, it truly struck me how much our society undervalues domestic work. Like, we don't value it at all.

My mum, who stayed at home until I was one and then went back to work two days a week, pretty much worked part-time while raising four kids and she has a strong view on this: 'I went to a party and people were talking about what they did and someone asked me and I replied, "I'm a mother, I look after my children." And then they said, "No, what do you actually do?" I was incensed. You're not "just" a stay-at-home-mum, you *are* a stay-at-home mum and, for me, I have the utmost respect for people who choose that.'

Dad piped up while Mum and I were having this chat. 'When asked what you do, people talk about a job or

occupation—mothering should be valued in the exact same way.'
It's probably fitting I mention here that Dad joked years ago
that the last of his three daughters to be married would pocket
$10,000. As a disincentive, so we could chase our dreams before
supposedly settling down. Ange always likes to remind him, 'I'm
not married yet!'

As I am finishing off this chapter, rather serendipitously, the
National Working Families Report is released. It finds two-thirds
of the 6289 working parents surveyed are struggling to care for
their physical and mental health due to the tension between work
and caring for kids. The majority were women, of course, who
said their biggest challenge was looking after their own physical
health and wellbeing. Societal pressures—the tangible stuff—play
a significant role in perpetuating our overwhelm. Mentally we feel
exhausted, guilty and completely and utterly unbalanced.

Changing cultural mindsets and unconscious attitudes is
extremely hard. It takes years, decades even—governments need
to step up and make policy changes, businesses need to do their
bit and all of us need to take stock inside our own workplaces and
homes. We have the facts and the stats: we know the mental health
struggle is real. Now we just need to get our smart heads together
and get on with redefining the struggle as it looks in each of our
lives. Even if it involves many hurried chats around the dinner
table—every conversation counts.

I thank the feminist gods that we've got people like Marian
Baird and Annabel Crabb championing our cause. Until we all
shift, the stress and overwhelm will go on and on. Either that, or
you pack up your life and move to Morocco . . . whatever gives you
a sense of true meaning in your life, I guess.

WISDOM
TANYA PLIBERSEK

Quick bio: Deputy Leader of the Australian Labor Party. Mum of three. Married. Just turned 50. Has been Member of Parliament for Sydney since 1998. Loves cooking and digital-free holidays.

Interview need-to-know: We sat down on a comfy couch in her sunny office in Sydney's Surry Hills. She was warm, calm and reassuring.

Q: You have a high-profile career, a successful husband and three kids—on the outside, you are the definition of 'having it all'. How do you manage it?

A: I feel incredibly lucky that I can combine work that I love and a family. Sometimes when things get stressful, I remind myself that I am lucky to be part of the generation which has these choices, but it does get pretty stressful. I just accept that there are two things in my life at the moment—family and work—and there's no time for anything else. It's really good if you can find the things that make you feel good and mix that in with family time—we were doing boxing training together; we go to the gym or bushwalking.

Q: You've talked about the importance of creating family rituals, tell me about that.

A: Someone once told me the three things you need to be happy are: someone to love, someone to love you back and something to look forward to. So, planning time to spend together is important. One of the things around Christmas is our family holiday and we go places where there is no phone or internet. A regular digital detox—even a weekend—is really healthy to get out and talk to each other.

Q: Can you share a time in your life when the juggle was absolutely real?

A: When Anna, now eighteen, was a baby, it was International Women's Day and we put out a press release the night before about the growing gender pay gap. I was doing radio interviews in the morning, and she had one of those nights where she had to sleep up on my shoulder, with reflux. All night, I'd been falling asleep sitting up. Michael was flying interstate early. I was feeding her through every interview and thinking, *It's so great, I've got it all!*

Q: Sometimes I wonder if we're honest enough with each other about our dark times—whether it be a baby, relationship breakdown or ageing parents. It must be hard on you travelling to Canberra all the time and leaving them behind.

A: I miss them a lot. It is a requirement of the job and there's always someone doing it much tougher. I never feel sorry for myself. I try to focus on the things to be grateful for—happiness and gratefulness are inextricably linked.

Q: When you didn't run for the Labor leadership in 2019, many women around me felt inspired by this. They felt you were saying it was okay not to put up your hand for the top job (often women feel guilty for not doing it in the name of feminism). What was the reaction at the time?

A: A mixed response. When you're making decisions about your family's wellbeing, you can't do that by anyone's rules other than your own. It just didn't feel right at that time. It's not saying that I'll never want to take on greater responsibilities in the future . . . I don't want women to think you can't balance a career and family life—you absolutely can—and I've been doing it for 21 years. It's not an all-or-nothing thing, you have to make your own judgements about how far you can go in that juggle for your own health and wellbeing. Most young men are also thinking this: how can we manage it in a healthier way?

Q: What do you feel are the most pressing issues for women when it comes to our health and wellbeing?

A: The two overwhelming issues for public policy are economic security and independence—we've got a pay and retirement income gap—and domestic violence. In the area of balancing work and family, the false notion of other people's perfect lives that is driven by social media is really toxic. If you're hard-working and a perfectionist by nature, the drive for unattainable excellence in every sphere in your life is not good—you have to be great at work, a perfect mother and have a beautifully decorated house and Instagrammable holidays.

Q: As I sit here and talk to you, I feel that perhaps balance is achievable after all, as you sound like you've nailed it . . .

A: It depends on your expectations, your definition. I think a lot of people put way too much pressure on themselves to do every element of their life perfectly. I am happy with the balance in my life . . . I love my job—I find it intellectually and emotionally rewarding. I have a happy home life, so those two things balance each other out—being able to move between work and home automatically gives me balance . . . But it doesn't mean I don't feel periods of intense stress. I just know that it's part of life.

'Once you understand what the mental load is, you become aware of it—you say, "Oh, that's the thing I can't turn off. That's the thing I feel, that's why I am so tired all the time, so overwhelmed, overworked and exhausted." Or "That's why I can't concentrate at work . . ."'

Leah Ruppanner, Associate Professor,
University of Melbourne

CHAPTER FIVE

THE PROBLEM THAT NOW HAS A NAME

There's a hush from the 130-odd women (and a few blokes) as Dr Libby Weaver walks swiftly down one of the aisles at the Kirribilli Club in Sydney to kick off her two-hour 'Overcoming Overwhelm: Getting to the Heart of Stress' event. It's bang on 7 p.m.

Dressed in jeans, a gleaming sequined T-shirt and a cool beige leather jacket, with her brown hair high in a slick pony, she looks nothing like your typical biochemist. But what do they look like anyway? Someone in a white coat, I guess. Dr Libby is not only an internationally acclaimed nutritional biochemist, she's also the bestselling author of twelve books—and looks like you, me, your friend, your neighbour, your barista, albeit healthier and glowier. Having notched up twelve years at uni, she is the right woman to give expert advice to sort out the jumble in your head. She is warm in her welcome.

Tonight's event is part of a 35-stop tour around Australia and New Zealand. Yes, there are a lot of stressed women (and some men) seeking advice and, no, I'm not surprised. I'm also here to get a clear visual of what a plethora of overwhelmed women look like. It's a wide range of women—from those dressed in Lululemon tights to stylish Cue suits, floaty floral dresses and distressed jeans—sitting on the wrought-iron chairs that you expect to find in these types of places. Women of every age, all with tired faces. In front of me, there's a mum with her daughter still in school uniform who is constantly checking social media on her phone. To my right is a woman, late thirties perhaps, who looks like she's wiping tears from her eyes while also reading her phone. On my other side is a twenty-something gym-goer, hair up in a messy topknot, who's already purchased three of Dr Libby's books from the makeshift book stand in the corner.

I've brought along Chloe, one of my best mates, who is as unbalanced as me. I picked her up from her gym around 6.30 p.m.—her husband is in New Zealand for work, and she 'had to' squeeze in a sweaty twenty-minute CrossFit workout after leaving her three kids with a babysitter. Tom is also away for work, so I'd left my three with our babysitter—the preschooler clinging to me and nearly ripping open the container of blueberries in my hand as I pried myself out of his arms and bolted out the front door. The blueberries, they're my dinner. There's one thing that binds us in this room: the modern-day juggle. The 'I'm so stressed, I'm so stressed' mantra that plays on repeat in our heads.

Dr Libby gets straight into it; she talks with a hint of worry in her voice. She is clear on how our body buckles under stress, how our self-talk perpetuates the cycle and, yes, how we can find a way out. Nearly two hours later, Chloe and I pack up our things. There is a queue of women eagerly waiting to buy Dr Libby's latest book, *The Invisible Load*, looking for more answers. We leave armed with pages of notes—I'll share more of those later.

Let's chat about your mental load

You and I could sit here and trade mental load lists for the rest of kingdom come, over a cup of tea or a bottle of wine. Nah, let's toast our lists with champagne—gives them much more punch.

During our first chat, Leah described the mental load to me as all of the thinking, planning, organisation and worry work. 'It's not just organisational tasks,' she said, 'but the remembering of what has to be done, what needs to be done that relates to the house and making sure the family is functioning. It's one of those things you inherently feel but don't realise it's draining you. Then, actually, once you understand what the mental load is, once you become aware of it—you say, "Oh that's the thing I can't turn off. That's the thing I feel, that's why I am so tired all the time, so overwhelmed, overworked and exhausted." Or "That's why I can't concentrate at work, I'm thinking about all the planning about school holidays or childcare."'

Whether it's organising the annual family camping trip, a catch-up with old schoolmates you haven't seen for yonks, contraception, or organising a birthday present for your partner's brother's child, you are the 'she-fault' option, the day-to-day manager of your household, kids or no kids. It's the nonstop minutiae of daily tasks and getting lost in the overwhelm of it all.

The mental load is not a single thing. It's like a million tiny pricks all at once, it's like always being jet lagged, or hungover, and you never feel clear-headed. The chatter and niggling in your head—it's like there are 345 tabs open all at once and you're constantly flicking between 344 of them from the moment you wake up to when you finally nod off to sleep. All day. Every day.

You with me on this? Thought so.

UK journalist Gemma Hartley penned a hard-hitting and fascinating book called *Fed Up,* published in 2018. I love her description of emotional labour and I want to share it with you: 'We lend an ear. We offer advice. We soothe egos and acknowledge the feelings of others while muting our own. We nod. We smile. We care. Perhaps most importantly, we do so without expecting any reciprocation, because emotional labour is women's work. We all know it.'

I believe most women will identify with this, and women without children should not be ejected from this conversation—we *all* feel overloaded. Overwhelm is a personal thing. Whether you're 25 or 45, everyone carries a mental load of sorts. It will change, mould, reshape and you'll redefine what it looks like, what it means, as you move through stages and are faced with unexpected situations like a relationship breakdown, losing your job, illness or tragedy. If you have kids, it feels like the mental load has an uncanny knack of hanging around like a bad smell, a reminder of all the shit you still need to do for yourself and those who depend on you. Then again, looking back to when I didn't have kids, my mental load often felt . . . heavy.

I work with Abbey. She's in her early twenties, and is always smiley and up-vibe when I walk into the office. In 2019, she wrote a piece for *whimn* titled 'We Need To Talk About The Mental Load of Living Solo', which reminded me that there are many different versions of a mental load, depending on your circumstances. My overwhelm is different to yours and is different to my sister's. Anyway, here's what Abbey said:

When you live by yourself, you live *with* yourself. Your home becomes an extension of your brain. And your thoughts, good or bad, rocket around the room with nothing to soften the blow.

Instead of walking through the door to one million happy distractions, it's just you. All the chaos of the day, plus dishes in the sink, bills to be paid, and not a single person to give you a hand or ask you how you are. There's surprisingly little downtime for a lifestyle that was pitched to be tranquil. Because silence and serenity are very different things. No one is relying on you, but you are also not relying on anyone.

This so-called invisible load has popped in and out of feminist theory for years. In 1983, the concept of 'emotional labour' was flagged to us (if you were born, that is) by American sociologist Professor Arlie Russell Hochschild in her book *The Managed Heart*. She called it out as the extra work some people take on to keep others in the group happy and healthy—a bit like air hosties whose job it is to be kind and friendly, to make everyone else onboard feel warm and fuzzy. A little over ten years later, in 1996, a US sociologist by the name of Susan Walzer (I am beginning to really dig these people) published a research paper called 'Thinking About The Baby', where she interviewed 23 couples with a new baby. She concluded that women do, in fact, carry more of the mental load, as it was predominantly the women who *first* noticed everything that needed to be done. In 2015, researchers picked up on Hochschild's research and looked at nurses of both genders—about 730 of them in a Midwestern hospital in the US. They found that women primarily carried more emotional labour in the workplace and men's 'privileged status' shielded them from having to perform it as frequently as women. That's the evidence right there: women carry an invisible load.

In 2017 a comic strip titled 'You Should've Asked'—by a French graphic artist known as Emma—gave it a name, and a collective 'OMG' could be heard around the Western world.

'The mental load means always having to remember,' the comic strip said, with all the to-remember things in cute thought bubbles. As Emma put it: 'The mental load is almost completely borne by women. It's permanent and exhausting work. And it's invisible.'

I love the title of this cartoon, don't you? 'You Should've Asked' also highlights our role as 'the manager'—like we're supposed to remember the fine print of the household runnings: whether it's bin night or school library day or when we're due for dinner at the in-laws'. Seriously, how easy is it to look in the fridge to check the milk supply, rather than asking the 'household manager'? Yet somehow, it's always the woman who knows when the lite white is running low and the almond milk is near to full.

Emma juggled being a mother with her job as a computer science engineer. It's kind of ironic that her side hustle—being an artist—gave her a global audience, because she captured the frustration of what generations of women had been trying to say: 'We're not born with an all-consuming passion for clearing tables, just like the boys aren't born with an utter disinterest for things lying around.' In short, genetics shouldn't define our roles on the home front.

> ➹ *If you haven't seen the comic strip, google it. It's mind-blowingly poignant and it really nails it; it's truthful, smart, emotive. It's also a bestselling book:* The Mental Load: A Feminist Comic. *Emma is sharp on including men in the discussion on how to improve things: when they say 'You should've asked', it merely confirms us as the she-fault parent, the doer-of-things.*

An article in *The New York Times*, 'What "Good" Dads Get Away With', went ultra-viral in 2019. Its author, Darcy Lockman, called the division of emotional labour/mental load 'one of the most important gender-equity issues of our time'. Columnists from Melbourne to Manchester to Minneapolis have all called it out as the next frontier of feminism.

Bring it on.

But wait. There's a problem. At the current rate of change, it might be another 75 years before there is parity between men and women when it comes to 'unpaid work'. Which includes all that shit we do. I don't want to wait that long—I don't want my daughter to be having these conversations with me in twenty years time, asking me why my generation let it happen.

I have so many questions about all of this. First and foremost (as Dr Lockman asked), why is this still happening?

Let's start by looking at why we do it to ourselves: why do we say yes and take on more than we know we can humanly handle? Why do we waste our valuable mental space on stuff that doesn't *really* matter? (A Pinterest-inspired colour-coded bookshelf, anyone?) Really, that's an hour of our time that could be devoted to stoking our wellbeing.

But, my friends, we are born into a society where women are still effectively the managers of household chores—'Household Management Project Leader', as Emma dubbed the role. The ones who have to remember everything. We are socialised to do it—the mental load is socialised along gender lines and, culturally, most of us accept it.

We also do it because we like a sense of control, as Jane Caro reminded me when we met, and power in our domain, our home. We like things done our way. Oh gosh, I do. The media doesn't help this whole scenario either—heard the phrase 'ad dad'? You know the handsome blokes who are called on in a crisis, but when it comes to putting on a nappy . . . Ha! No idea. He'd have more luck on a *Ninja Warrior* set. The *Community Responses to Gender*

Portrayals in Advertising report from RMIT University and Women's Health Victoria found that gender stereotyping is rife in advertising. Too often, Dad's out kicking the footy while Mum— portrayed as a sexy housewife, of course—is mopping the floor. Yes, people, this *still* happens in advertising in 2020! Worryingly, the report found we are so desensitised to this that we don't even complain about it.

This makes me wonder what a good mother looks like these days. Am I a good mother? Am I a good worker? Now I'm worried. It looks like the requirements for being a good mother and a good worker are simply incompatible.

'In an era where "good" mothers are those who are unequivocally invested in our children and "good" women always have a squeaky clean home and fresh biscuits on display, the mental load is on steroids, requiring women's constant attention," Leah told the ABC's brilliant podcast *Ladies, We Need To Talk*. 'The mental and physical load is just too high. But by assuming the managerial role in the home, women are absolving other family members of this exhausting work. For married couples, this means men have more mental space to plan for work and to decompress in leisure. For many women, housework and the mental load are cast as ways to love and care for the family. Yet, questions of equity are important here, especially if women's absorption of the mental load and the managerial role are at the expense of their employment, sleep, leisure and health.'

She's bang-on, you know.

My neighbour Jen reminded me of this: 'You give birth to a child and your wings are clipped. In terms of your life, you fly but not so high.'

🔊 'You don't compare a Ferrari to a Ford, so don't follow a young 21-year-old who loves protein shakes on Instagram and expect to feel great. For me, I want the real life from the mummas: we need to show the juggle, the bum wiping, the dirty floors and the whole 'ships in the night' relationship reality. We need to see the whole damn picture. Because I dare say the women that are rocking it 100 billion-fold often have hubby at home, or a nanny, or a crazy amount of family help. Or, they're so close to burnout that I want to jump through the phone screen and catch them as they fall.'—*Stace*

The care factor

I decide to call Dr Rebecca Huntley to ask her about all this. She knows exactly what we're collectively feeling, as she talks to hundreds and hundreds of Australian women every year. She's one of Australia's leading social researchers and an author with degrees in law and film studies and a PhD in gender studies. Rebecca knows her stuff. I've seen her presentations many times throughout my career and she always impresses me, juggling her busy schedule with her husband while raising three kids. I catch her just as she is about to pick up her kids from school. I'm in the car, again. Worryingly, she adds another element into the mental load conundrum.

'There is a lot of tension and discussion about how we change this . . . we are still right in the middle of really struggling to work out not so much whether these changes need to happen, but how we deal with the consequences,' she explains. 'One thing I find is that women, after a while, find the constant fight with their partner—for whatever equality looks like to them—pretty tiring.

So, they decide to work around them. They say, "I'm raising my sons and daughters to help me out." Or, "I'm working more to earn more to get things outsourced." Or they make a decision to just live with it, which can be hard, and every now and then it gets chronic when nothing is working in the house.

'Behaviour change is a difficult thing . . . often women feel like they can't have another fight and that's where fatigue and stress come in because they're doing absolutely everything. I see women in their fifties when their marriages have broken down because they're sick of it. Men re-partner quickly because they're lonely, but women don't because they don't want to clean up after another dude.'

There is so much to think about here—how could I change what I do around the house? I walk downstairs to pop some bread into the toaster (I have a hankering for toast with butter and jam—don't judge me for being unhealthy) and automatically start stacking the dishwasher. My eldest son, who is buttering his own toast, turns to me and—I kid you not—says, 'You're always doing everything, Mum. You never stop.' The second son pipes up. 'Yeah, Mum. Why do you need to do everything at the same time?'

Tears prick my eyes. I draw a deep breath. I turn to both of my sons, crouching down to reply, 'I do everything because I love you, because I care, because I want your lives to run smoothly, to be less stressful and fun. It makes me happy, joyful even, to know you have a great day because I've helped you.' I might sound like an 'ad mum', but I mean it.

As I carry my toast back into our makeshift office, I remind myself, too, that I get immense satisfaction from helping them. It gives me a sense of purpose and brings meaning to my life. In fact, the same goes for every other important person in my life—my husband, parents, siblings, friends, workmates, and even my next-door neighbour.

Actually, Dr Libby pointed this exact thing out to me, too: we do it because we care. She's right: we as women are deeply caring individuals and if we stopped doing what we do, we believe the people around us would suffer. But would they really? Maybe sometimes but not all the time. Either way, we suffer instead. 'It's as if we've put on a backpack and filled it with rocks,' explains Dr Libby. 'We walk around with it on and we really don't know what the rocks are. We have beliefs about ourselves, as we're not born with our personality or identity, we create it.'

I keep coming back to the Jean Hailes research—we worry, we can't sleep, we have no time for us, we have mind blanks, we feel helpless. (Go back to page 26 if you need a reminder.) The relentless full-time job that is the mental load is a major contributing factor to our lack of mental wellbeing. It's yet another thing fuelling our exhaustion. Our stress. Our guilt. Our anxiety. Our overwhelm. We have less time to focus on our physical selves (have you *ever* done a yoga class without thinking about your to-do list?), and not enough time to examine our emotional or spiritual headspace. Our mental load nibbles away at the valuable time that could be spent on our hobbies or simply relaxing outside in the sunshine with a good book.

The mental load many of us carry today—I'm pondering my own backpack overflowing with rocks—is more detrimental to our wellbeing than it ever has been.

> 'My husband and I have had some big chats about the mental load and now that he understands what the concept actually means, there have been some real improvements in our house. Sometimes to the point where I question myself: "Am I dropping the ball?" Then I have to remind myself, "No, this is probably what a 50/50 household actually is"—it just feels so foreign.'—*Lizie*

The social media conundrum

I want to take a moment to chat about social media and the role it plays in all this. Don't we know it. If you're one of the, dare I say, smarter folk who don't buy into it—or if you're having a momentary digital detox (well done, you)—then skip along to the next chapter. If not, stick with me here.

Don't get me wrong, there are many wonderful benefits of social media. I use it. I like it. It makes you laugh and inspires you, and allows you to reconnect with old friends, build side hustles, rally a country to vote 'yes', discover a nifty new handyman, introduce new words into the Zeitgeist (FOMO, anyone?) and let's not forget the gift that is Celeste Barber.

Really, I can't live without it. However, I can't help but notice the increasing number of studies linking its consumption to poorer mental health. It is fifteen years since Facebook first launched, so it's only now we're getting a solid grasp on its true impact on our mental health. In a nutshell, studies have linked social media to anxiety, depression, loneliness, lack of sleep, cyber-bullying, narcissism, poor body image, decreased physical activity and addiction. Yes, one study saw parallels between regular social media users and drug addicts.

In 2017, Facebook itself publicly admitted that social media can have a negative impact on our noggins. 'In general, when people spend a lot of time passively consuming information— reading but not interacting with people—they report feeling worse afterwards,' it said in a statement. Sure, all this is amplified in teens and young women as it's now woven into the fabric of their lives. In terms of us—you, me and the women around us—what I worry about most is its impact on our self-talk, self-image and self-esteem. When everyone is showing their highlight reels, often through a fairytale filter, it's sometimes hard to see your own life as good enough. Whether it's fitness, food, social functions, health, motherhood or holidays, this comparison environment also drives our desire for competition. The women you follow can look like they have it all (and more!), but it's a distorted view of what their lives are *really* like. Influencers are first to say, 'Come on, but everyone knows it's not real life, it's only a snapshot.' Of course we know that. I mean, we don't see people when they first wake up, when their marriage is falling apart, or when their latest Tinder date is a douche. But we too often forget this when we're mindlessly scrolling for the twentieth time that day. Funny how when you're bored, or tired, you reach for the phone and scroll Facebook. Join the club.

There's a study I came across a while ago that I often reference when talking about this stuff on TV. It found that even if you're generally happy in life, if your body image is healthy and your self-esteem mostly intact, social media can still have a negative effect on your thoughts. It comes down to being human and our fundamental drive to compare ourselves to others—we do this to evaluate our own decisions, regulate our emotions and, of course, find inspiration. You see, normally we do this within our friendship circles—people we see day-to-day—so we are privy to their struggles, too. The problem with social media is we're only seeing the happiest and most successful side of everyone, so you're comparing your realistic self to someone else's idealised online self, which can then be detrimental to wellbeing and self-evaluation. Facebook, Instagram and Twitter are absolutely compounding our feelings of overwhelm, mental exhaustion and stress, further fuelling life's imbalance.

It's not just social media. In today's society, we're constantly bombarded with images (I'm also pointing the finger at the media and magazines—yes, the stuff I create) reminding us that we're not good enough. These ubiquitous messages reinforce unattainable expectations of our appearance and lifestyle. And there's another downside: they expose our vulnerabilities and perpetuate our insecurities. We participate in social media to show our worth. We lap it up to feed our worth. No wonder it can make us feel pretty crap. Research does suggest that our brains gravitate towards the negative, thanks to the fight or flight response that our cave-ancestors relied on. We click on that news story that will make us feel scared, angry or sad to make sure we know how to protect ourselves if it ever does happen.

When Dr Libby is in Sydney for her 'Overcoming Overwhelm' talk, I meet up with her in a chic hotel lobby in Sydney. She's from South Queensland, you see. Dr Libby has really been banging on about our daily life battleground for years—apart from her great books, she's done an informative TEDx Talk titled 'The Pace of Modern Life Versus Our Cavewoman Biochemistry'—another thing to add to your to-watch list. (Eek, sorry.)

She tells me she has started to get *really* worried about the increase in stress-related health issues she's seeing—digestive systems gone haywire, hormone imbalances, body image angst and the like. As she talks me through the research for her latest book, *The Invisible Load: A guide to overcoming stress and over-whelm,* I am nodding in furious agreement. She is talking about *me,* and what I've observed in friends, work colleagues, women on discussion boards and Facebook feeds. In the late teens and early twenties, she found, the two top stressors for women are Instagram and body image. 'Then, it all shifts from, say, 26 and upwards, and it becomes overflowing emails, to-do lists that are never done.

They describe the modern-day juggling act of managing work and a home, raising children, paying the bills, paying the mortgage, partners.'

I leave the lobby and jump in an Uber to go home—to dinner, kids, homework and anything else that life wants to throw at me tonight. I feel a bit despondent. It makes me wonder: where the hell is wellness when we really need it?

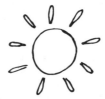

'The older I'm getting, the more I'm realising that my goal is far less work-oriented and more about a calm, chilled-out life. My Instagram's not going to look very fun this weekend, but god, my soul feels happier.'

Carrie Bickmore, TV host

CHAPTER SIX # #SUPERWOMAN, WE HAVE A PROBLEM

You should have seen the lists I made for my wedding. Come to think of it, I couldn't have shown you all of them because I was ticking off and rewriting them constantly in my Excel spreadsheet. There were about fifteen on one count, including dressmaker options, bridesmaid tasks and ceremony to-do lists.

Planning a wedding is a bit like the Brexit kerfuffle: vexing. I'm sure if you've gotten hitched, you're with me on this. My brother and sister-in-law eloped to Florence, Italy, and I'm seriously envious of that. Tom and I got married in Far North Queensland and, because we hailed from way down south, the spreadsheets were my way of keeping control of my stress. Guests had to travel, so I wanted them to fly home from the wedding extravaganza saying to each other, 'Holy hell, that was amazing!'

Mind you, I had this 'I-can-do-it-all' feeling—that one where you're channelling Superwoman, except she's nowhere in sight to actually help you out. I also had this messed-up mindset that no one else could do it the way I wanted it, not even Tom. It had to be perfect, no, *perfectly* perfect. The curse of perfectionism in full swing.

All this leaves me wondering, have we raised the bar so high that it is becoming our own mental undoing?

The curse of self-sabotage

I have a few questions for you. How many of these statements have you told yourself in the past week or so? Please tweak so they fit your life circumstances. Okay, here goes . . .

- I am crap at cooking myself/partner/kids/flatmate healthy food.
- Oh man, I feel so guilty for not calling 'insert best friend's name here' this week.
- I don't spend enough time with my kids.
- My house isn't clean enough.
- I don't know how much maternity leave to take without jeopardising my career.
- I feel terrible. I said I'd cook this cake for my friend's baby shower, but now I can't be arsed.

Honestly, I've recited different versions of these—and thousands more—too often in my days. If I examine those statements in isolation, I wonder why I was beating myself up.

We try to be superwoman to all the people around us, we comment with the hashtag #superwoman whenever we see an influencer doing *everything* and we fully lap up anything superwoman-y—T-shirts, cards and cute coffee mugs—and why shouldn't we? I do love how feminism has sparked new life into this superhero character; what I *don't* love is how we hold up women to these higher standards.

The expectations we hold for ourselves—and the ones society places on women—are fuelling our mental exhaustion in many ways. Conscious or unconscious, that's just how it is. #Superwoman is a mythical status that is too hard to achieve. The expectations build up little by little, without you even realising. It's a heavy burden we all carry, yet we all buy into it. I mean, do you really need to spend an extra hour before your friend's barbecue making that Donna Hay quinoa and goat's cheese salad when you could grab an equally tasty one from Woolies in five minutes? (I do love Donna Hay, but on Saturday morning when all hell is breaking loose—hello, Woolies!)

It means we end up doing more than perhaps we really need to—around the house, in our work lives, in our social circles—and this can eat into the valuable time we could otherwise be using to focus on our own wellbeing. If you don't have kids, you might put in extreme hours at the gym, food prep all day Sunday for your week ahead or slave over a work presentation—all because that's what we think we should be doing. If you have kids, then this new domesticity movement is in overdrive as mothers are required to grow their own veggies, raise chickens, organise their pantries with military-like precision, colour block their bookshelves, knit their kids' socks and . . . and move to Byron Bay.

It's the 'cult of intensive motherhood' that runs on guilt, as Brigid Schulte calls it in *Overwhelmed*.

I know that so-called impostor syndrome fuels this vicious cycle, especially in the workplace. We feel like we're just not good enough. I'm absolutely sure you've heard of this term, coined in 1978 (yes, it's been around that long) by two psychologists, Pauline Clance and Suzanne Imes. They called it a psychological pattern where you think you're a fraud, doubt your accomplishments and believe you don't deserve your achievements. It can be distinguished by six key factors: the impostor cycle, the need to be special, fear of failure, guilt over success, identifying with the characteristics of superwoman and inability to accept praise. When our expectations are too high, of course we are going to doubt our own achievements and that, dear reader, is emotionally exhausting. It's the natural enemy of balance and wellness, don't you think . . . ?

'How very many layers we operate on, and how very many influences we receive from our minds, our bodies, our histories, our families, our cities, our souls and our lunches!' wrote Elizabeth Gilbert in *Eat, Pray, Love.*

True that.

Society, what do you expect?

My go-to sociologist, Leah, shared a study with me that illustrates it's not just our own expectations, but also wider society's, that feed into this superwoman aspiration. She and her colleagues randomly assigned 327 men and 295 women one photo of a messy room and another photo of a tidier room. Then they told participants that the rooms in the photos belonged to either Jennifer or John. All participants equally rated the level of mess, which debunked any theory that only women are biologically programmed to see mess. Leah and her colleagues then asked the participants to rate Jennifer and John's character—how respons-ible, hardworking, neglectful, considerate and likeable they were—based on the cleanliness of their room. They also asked, 'What if your boss or friends dropped by unexpectedly? What would they think?' And that's where things got interesting, Leah told me. The participants responded differently depending on whether the room belonged to a male or female. They had higher expectations of cleanliness for Jennifer compared with John.

Here's the kicker: they not only saw Jennifer as less competent, they judged her character more harshly than John's. What the *hell?!*

Leah says we see mess and get into a cycle of 'fear-cleaning'. I know I do. Frantically running or stomping around your house, cleaning up because your friends are coming over. Jostling cupboards jammed with too much stuff shut. I mean, do your friends really care if the cushions aren't straight? If there is a dead cockroach on the carpet? If Lego covers the floor of your kid's room? Or your partner's clothes are on the bedroom floor? Just make sure you have the Ecoya candles burning. Ha!

But now you can see why we do it, right? We want to meet our own, our friends', and society's high expectations of what it means to behave like a good, responsible, caring, kind and got-it-all-together woman.

If only they knew what was happening on the inside . . .

There was a cartoon by Michael Leunig in 2019 that blew up in the media. You know the guy? His drawing showed a woman, fingers all over her mobile, pushing a pram. But the baby wrapped in blue had fallen out and was lying behind her on the ground. In his cunning caption underneath, he implied the mum loved social media more than her baby.

This caused a stir in feminist circles (particularly within Clementine Ford's following) and on mummy Facebook groups. Rightly so. It was a shining example of the shaming that happens when women don't meet society's expectations.

When I saw it, I thought, *Eff-off.* F-the-effety-f-off. Do you know what my morning has been like? My day? My life? No, instead you're passing judgement on my social media habits that you, dear older white man, know nothing about.

And let's take a moment to think about Meghan Markle. You know those stories about the malicious Duchess of Sussex destroying the Royal Family that you feel guilty for clicking on, but do anyway? Do you click on ones of Prince Harry with equal gusto? Probably not. We all mum-shame even if we hate it. We also fat-shame, slut-shame, career-shame, single-shame and so on.

We judge. Criticising another woman is a shameful act in itself. And if she doesn't meet our expectations then we shame her even more.

Dr Grant Blashki, a GP and lead clinical adviser at Beyond Blue, sees a large number of women for mental health issues who are grappling with a complex tangle of stressors. He told the *Sydney Morning Herald* that he considers the social expectations on young women to be very high: 'I'll often come home at the end of a busy day in clinic and say to my wife, "It's not easy being a young woman these days".'

What happens when we don't meet our own expectations? Guilt, shame, worry and stress. Too often we judge ourselves more harshly than we judge other people, and studies show that a third of women buckle under so-called perfectionism—the deep belief that you're never quite good enough because of your own high and unrealistic expectations. You know, because everything has to be #perfect. Often when we're stressed, our default is self-criticism. We dwell on things we may or may not have done or said, but compare that to the typical man's response. In many ways they, as my husband would say, just get on with it. I say, 'Oh, but I could have done so much better.' Tom's response is, 'But that's good enough.' So, when you want everything to be perfect, you can see the cycle you get into.

This, my friend, can lead to feelings of worry, sadness, anger, anxiety and depression. Yes, perfectionism depletes wellbeing.

'As a woman, making an effort isn't good enough, because we are constantly bombarded with the message that we need to be perfect,' writes Gemma Hartley in *Fed Up*. 'At every turn, advertising and media remind us that if only we try a *little* harder, if we stretch a *little* farther, perfection is within our reach.'

The house a little cleaner, our wardrobe a little more organised, our body a little fitter, a little skinner, a little healthier, our bank account a little richer, a little . . . *sigh.* It's relentless, day in and day out and it's *exhausting.* And then comes the guilt . . . because if you've done your best, you've given it your all . . . then, what's left? Not time for you, not time to focus on your mental wellbeing. You just can't take a break. You feel guilty for sitting still and doing nothing, even for a minute. You beat yourself up for your lack of productivity when, really, unproductiveness can be one of the best remedies for being overwhelmed.

There is no such thing as a #superwoman, so let's stop telling people there is, and instead ask women if they are okay.

Often I wonder if all the jumble in our heads and the feelings it perpetuates come back to us not being honest enough with each other—about our internal and external struggles. We don't talk enough about life being overwhelming; we're scared to reveal our shortcomings, our vulnerabilities and ongoing insecurities. We live in isolation a lot of the time, and I don't count Facebook threads as true human connection (well, only sometimes). We're not yelling over our back fences like we did circa 1962, putting our hands up to pick up the kids from school or asking to borrow a dress for that thirtieth on Saturday night. When was the last time you left a lasagne on someone's front doorstep? Now I know we all *want* to do it, we think about it and we do it sometimes, but perhaps not enough. Then again, how can we do it when we're so overloaded with our own life stuff . . . and so the vicious cycle of the modern-day juggle continues.

I'm often reluctant to tell women without kids how bloody hard it can be after you push out your first one. I want them to approach it all with a sense of hope. I don't want to be an exhausted, career-goal shattered, burnt-out mother whining about how crappy life is because . . . there are good bits and great bits! It's just there is a hell of a lot of shit, too. Before I had kids, I used to hear this whingeing and somehow default to 'But that won't happen to me. It will be different for me'.

My trusty feminist ally Jane Caro talks about this too. 'There is such pressure for mothers to talk about it all being amazing, fulfilling, and how everything is amazing and wonderful,' she says. 'No, that's not how it is. It's snotty and shitty and you're always tired. And the drudgery . . . We have decided that life is controllable and if you only tried hard enough, you could have a perfect life like that person on social media.'

> ✒ 'I used to get a lot of pressure to have kids in my early thirties, but our life is our own personal journey and other people's expectations should not become the expectations you have of yourself.'—*Ange*

If only I had the time . . .

All this stuff going on in our heads . . . I mean, if only we had time to sift through it all. If only we had time to make sense of our emotions, our feelings, our spiritual side. If only we had time to *ourselves* to nurture our wellbeing.

We ran a story in *Women's Health* that always pops into my head when I'm mentally weighing up what's more deserving of my time—the gym or staying back at work that extra hour. Or perhaps Netflix. Actually, no, it's when I am screaming to myself, *I don't have time!* The story was hooked on a study of 4000 Americans who were asked what they valued more: time or money, and also how happy they were. Not surprisingly, 65 per cent valued money but the ones who valued time were generally happier. Married people and parents valued their time more highly, understandably, as did older people. Parents especially cherished their time, yet also felt their time was stolen from them.

Where does the time go? The days, the years? Whether you're 25 or 45, most of us feel more pressed for time than ever—to meet work deadlines, to apply for that next job, to tick off your travel bucket list or house to-do list. Most of us feel utterly and exhaustingly time-poor day in and day out.

> ➤ *Remember, the words you tell yourself (and others) matter. They carry power. Ask yourself this: is saying 'I don't have time' a B.S. excuse for not wanting to do something? It's about scheduling your priorities. (More on this in Part Two.)*

There's a worldwide army of science boffins studying the whole concept of time, looking at areas like technology (which is supposed to make life easier and save us time), work structures, and, of course, parenting. Clearly some time-wasting is of our own doing, er, social media mindless scrolling, anyone? Interestingly, parents spend twice as much time with their children today than 50 years ago and, yes, women put in more of this time than men. Time studies have confirmed working mothers are the most time-poor humans walking the planet, weighed down by 'task density'. That's one way to describe it, I guess! Not only that, our time off is much more fragmented than that of men. Say, for example, you're on holidays and sitting by the pool reading, but you're also the one who's still got one eye on the kids or you're the one thinking about which restaurant you'll eat at later that night.

This kind of study also begs the obvious question: how do we, and how does society, value a woman's time compared to a man's time? Do we value it as equal? I think not. How often have you been privy to friends, mothers, mothers-in-law fawning over the time a bloke spends working on a project, preparing dinner or driving the kids around on a weekend? This, again, feeds back into our 14 per cent gender pay gap, the undervaluing of domestic work and so on . . . actually, all the gaps we are still fighting to close and which we're now rallying men to step up to help with.

It reminds me of the New Zealand-born economist Marilyn Waring, who was arguing feminist economics back in 2000, and made a valid point. She was discussing how to include unpaid labour in gross domestic product (GDP) and rather than using economic activity, which renders all the domestic work invisible, she suggested using time—it's the one investment we all share. Time is the perfect equaliser—we all have the same number of hours in a day and it's up to us—yes, *you*—to shuffle through your priorities and choose how you use them. I get it, this is easy to say, harder to practise. I mean, where do you find time to think about how you can find more time in your already time-stretched day? Who has the time to even think about time?

I can't help but wonder whether our value of time in the Western world leaves us with little time to just . . . be. Our lack of time is at the root of our overwhelm—we have no time for mental space to regroup, to recentre, to self-reflect, to sort through our mental mess. To remind ourselves what living a rich and mean-ingful life actually looks like—off the screens, out of our own heads, away from our to-do lists.

It's quite simple, really: we just want to find more mental space in our lives. I'm just not sure how to do that.

⏰ 'I find the happier I am, the more time there is for me because I want to make the time.'—*Stace*

Living like this is making us sick

The #superwoman tag broke me not so long ago. It literally made me sick. It's only now as I am writing this chapter—processing the gravity of the relentless, unforgiving thoughts in our heads—that I've realised this direct correlation. I would literally crawl into bed at the end of each day, bones aching, soul depleted, comforting myself in my soft, white cotton sheets. I would struggle to sleep as thoughts swirled around my head. But it was my body that carried the evidence, as it so often does when you're mentally burnt out and physically fried. For me, I broke out in head-to-toe, face included, psoriasis. (Randomly, Kim Kardashian also suffers from psoriasis and is vocal about her struggles, which makes me feel a bit better. Granted, it's the only thing we have in common.)

In recounting this, I am mindful that I have not suffered significant trauma like a divorce, the death of a child, addiction or a cancer diagnosis. The enormity of these life challenges abso-lutely supersedes anything I might have gone through—my stress is pretty tame in that respect. My health suffered simply due to mental and physical exhaustion, but I was so busy I didn't have time to notice until it was too late.

It was footy season, and Tom was working six to seven days a week. The kids were waking up throughout the night and I'd taken the three of them away five out of the past six weekends for various extended family commitments—you know, weddings and parents' birthdays. I was working part-time, full-time catering to everyone's emotional needs and running the household.

A vomiting virus ripped through said household, followed by tonsillitis . . . and I fell apart.

I went to see a nutritionist to sort out this sore and embarrassing skin thing. She diagnosed a leaky gut (confirmed via one of the most disgusting, self-inflicted ways—divvying up your poo into vials and posting it off for testing. Just gross). While recommending various remedies—no dairy, no gluten for a month—she kindly reminded me that with all my mental chatter about my body's deficiencies, I wasn't taking into account that my body had carried and fed three children in five years. No easy feat. This obvious assessment was surprisingly reassuring to hear. Much more palatable than the fact that giving up my latte addiction would cure my skin woes. Mind you, I cut back the coffee, quit the dairy, logged quality sleep (thanks Fitbit) and my psoriasis mostly cleared up.

Stress is such an individual, subjective thing, as Dr Ginni Mansberg, my go-to GP and author of *The M Word: How to thrive in menopause* (FYI: it's a great book), reminds me. Dr Ginni was the original GP at *Women's Health* and nowadays we often end up together in the green room before *Sunrise*. She tells me stress can be a strange one to study as it's hard to objectively measure. Some of us are genuinely stressed, whereas others are just plain busy. I find it bothersome how interchangeable the words have become. When you're stressed, it absolutely consumes your mind and body. Busy? It's a bit kinder on them both. But I agree that it's still important we validate every woman's individual struggle with it.

Every expert I spoke to agreed with Dr Ginni's take on stress. Even though we know there are many displaced women and children around the world, it's still okay to feel your own struggles. It's not a competition. Dr Ginni warns, though, that sometimes it can be 'a battle of the stress heroes'. Two women can report a similar level of stressful feelings, with one saying, 'My boss is such a bitch' and the other saying, 'Oh, to have a job'.

The physiological outcome can vary, too. Dr Ginni sees women who are beyond stressed, not sleeping, at risk of losing their jobs, whose cortisol levels—the hormone our body releases to respond to stress—are normal. Yet, other women, who are not coping and are exhausted, with no mental bandwidth left, have had cortisol levels higher than the Himalayas. Dr Ginni worries, too, about the increase in young women suffering social media stress.

In all the studies I've come across, women consistently report higher stress levels than men and, in turn, are more prone to burnout due to their modern-life juggle. I'll share the results of just one study. In 2016, researchers at the University of Cambridge reviewed over 1200 published studies about anxiety, and found that women are twice as likely as men to suffer from severe stress and anxiety. Some experts have even labelled it the 'stress gap'— just another gap to add to our ever-growing, feminist to-eradicate list. Sure, hormones, brain chemistry and coping strategies come into play (that is, how we tend to ruminate on that bad Bumble date versus how fast he moves on) but, overall, we feel it more. It's true, too, that stress peaks at different times in our lives—age 35 to 44 is when women's stress is shown to peak.

So, what happens to your body under stress? And to what extent are modern-day stressors chipping away at our health and wellbeing? This is something Dr Libby is big on; remember, she is a biochemist after all. When I asked her about this during our chat in the hotel lobby, she gave me a long, science-y, yet heartfelt answer. Here are the bits you'll find most relevant.

When a woman gets the message 'I am stressed' (the speed of life today being the main stressor), that message to her body triggers her adrenal glands to pump out a flood of stress hormones, like adrenalin and cortisol. Then, her body is all action stations thanks to our cavewoman fight or flight response. She's ready to run, baby. Her heart pumps, blood pressure rises, muscles flex, breath quickens—her senses are on high alert. Live in this state, like so many of us do, and some common symptoms of high cortisol are: a decrease in muscle mass and a change in body fat distribution. Where? You guessed it, your middle and back, which Dr Libby often refers to as 'a back verandah'.

> *Did you ever watch the* Kath & Kim *episode where they called the 'flaps' under a woman's arms 'fadoobadas'? It was* funny. *Yes, they're also known as bat wings, bingo wings or tuckshop lady arms and, by 30, we all have them. Come on, let's flap them together now.*

'A woman who is stressed then thinks she needs to diet, and what she's not seeing is that the body responds to the messages we give it,' Dr Libby says. 'We wake up and think of our to-do list and the 65 things we didn't get done yesterday that we need to pack into today. Then we go to work and there's 400 unopened emails. We're overwhelmed so we get a coffee, and there's more adrenalin across the day and we do it every day—it's a constant and relentless output of stress hormone and it's a massive change for us as modern women. We hardly ever produced it in cavepeople times, or if we did, it was in spikes, and then it was gone. The consistent output of adrenalin leads to inflammation and so then our body produces more cortisol because it's an anti-inflammatory. It has its own consequences: it breaks down your muscles, slows metabolism, increases body fat and messes with your body's ability to regulate glucose, so you crave more sugar, you're at greater risk of type 2 diabetes and that predisposes you to autoimmune diseases.'

Stress is linked to a long list of physical health issues, but most importantly to our mental wellbeing, as both Dr Libby and Dr Ginni agree—sleep deprivation is a fundamental sign that your body is in full-blown stress mode. As Dr Ginni says, 'Sleep has an enormous impact on your resilience, every day.'

As I chat to both Dr Ginni and Dr Libby about our lack of balance and our increasingly stress-filled lives, there is a real concern in their voices—an urgency for action. They genuinely worry that the modern-day juggle is harming our wellbeing.

Social researcher whiz Dr Rebecca Huntley has seen this firsthand in her interviews: 'I constantly see men and women struggle with these issues, and one of the consequences for women is a building up of resentment over time which can manifest itself in different ways, such as impacts on their health.'

I asked Dr Libby whether we're at a crisis point. 'I think it was at crisis ages ago and it's just gotten worse,' she says. 'It's every-where. I speak in regional areas and it's there. Sure, in Sydney or Melbourne or capital cities there is more intensity but fundament-ally it's the same thing. I'm trying to slow it down, if you like, as a lot of people just accept it when they don't like it—the pace of life, the stress—they feel powerless to change it and they feel trapped.'

Trapped is a word that comes up a lot when I speak to my friends, women at the school gate or during my lunch break. There is no way out, no light at the end of the breakneck speed tunnel and if we keep going at this pace, not only will our mental health suffer but our marriages, friendships and lives will fall apart and we'll pass all this anxiety onto our kids. We are mentally falling apart, little by little.

Something *has* to change . . . oh, that's right, we have a remedy! We have wellness . . .

WISDOM
FIFI BOX

Quick bio: A long-time radio superstar, heard on Melbourne's Fox FM. TV presenter (her bubbly self pops up on *The Project*). Mum to Trixie Belle and Daisy Belle. All-round cool chick.

Interview need-to-know: Fifi and I have shared seats in *Sunrise*'s make-up room (she was their weather presenter turned entertainment reporter circa 2009), shared lunches in New York City and had a shared struggle with the pregnancy condition hyperemesis gravidarum. Our chat happens over Instagram DM, as you do . . .

Q: How do you cope when you're overwhelmed with work?

A: When I'm overwhelmed in life (which seems to be all the time!) I immediately stop what I'm doing and breathe. This break is important to take the pressure down and give me some space in my head to sort things out, and then prioritise.

Q: How do you sift through it then?

A: I grab a pen and physically write down a list of everything I'm dealing with, things that are overwhelming me or need to be done. I find once my mind is calmed—it's like detangling a piece of string—life is far more manageable.

Q: Do you think balance is B.S.?

A: I believe in life balance because I know I suffer if I don't have it. I love being a mum and being with my children is my main love and priority, but I am a happier and more present mum if I find time to shift my focus temporarily to work. Similarly, the time spent on my career is more focused and enriched because I am happy having spent quality time with my girls. I get great satisfaction from working, and then when I put my mum hat back on, I rush back to the girls with excitement and energy that I may not have had if I had not left the house.

Q: How has motherhood changed you?

A: Motherhood has brought me more joy than I ever thought was possible. I have always been very career oriented and driven to succeed professionally, but when I had my children I achieved a sense of fulfilment I'd never felt before—my cup was finally full and nothing else mattered. Everything now has perspective.

'The minute the phrase "having it all" lost favor among women, wellness came in to pick up the pieces. It was a way to reorient ourselves—we were not in service to anyone else, and we were worthy subjects of our own care.'

Taffy Brodesser-Akner, *The New York Times Magazine*

CHAPTER SEVEN

THE WELLNESS SOLUTION

I've always had an intrinsic desire to feel healthy and well—I often wonder if it's just part of my DNA, like yours, I'm guessing. So the role of founding editor of *Women's Health* was my dream job. It was 2007 and health was still seen as a cure for illness rather than a lifestyle. Australia was the first country to launch the magazine outside the US.

I was deputy editor of *Cosmopolitan* when I applied. I would help rally our magazine team to run Sydney's City2Surf, I raced to step classes during my lunch breaks, went on skiing holidays and drank vegetable-choked smoothies all in the name of health (my trusty hangover cure, too). Mind you, I'm sure having a professional athlete as a partner also helped haul my butt off the couch and outside for a run.

The day I started at *Women's Health* was a momentous time. The Saturday before, Tom had skippered his AFL team, the Geelong Cats, to their first premiership in 44 years. And what a weekend of marvellous mayhem that was. Sigh. I flew back to Sydney late Sunday night and fronted up to my new office on Monday. (Sidenote: we survived long distance for three years before Tom moved to Sydney upon his footy retirement.)

No one was quite sure how triumphant this health magazine for women was going to be. I mean, *Men's Health*, with their buff cover hunks did pretty well, so we were confident a women's version wouldn't be too far behind. But we didn't expect to outsell them on our second issue.

Back then, the only gym chains for women were Fitness First and Fernwood, Lululemon was a thought in founder Chip Wilson's mind and quinoa didn't exist in our vocab let alone sit on the shelves of Coles. The word 'wellness' was only mentioned when people referred to hippies living in Nimbin, that place not far from Byron Bay. It's sobering to remember that it wasn't so long ago that wellness was actually still woo-woo.

I remember doing the rounds of advertising agencies in those first few years. I would stand up in front of a room full of upstarts and try to convince them that their client should sink $20K, $50K, $70K into our brand. People would stare at me blankly, like fitness was for freaks, and many didn't have a clue what wellness actually meant. Our main wins were with people who got it, those who ran next to me on the treadmill. Since I left that gig at the end of 2016, wellness has exploded—it's a new religion—and everyone from celebrities to social media's cool kids to kickass business leaders wants in. Me too.

A short history of the rapid rise of wellness

Wellness. Go on, say it out loud. *Welllllnessss.* The word alone evokes a kind of calming energy, doesn't it? In my mind, I imagine a totally serene me. Whatever that looks like—it's a rare sight these days. Before we delve deep into the world of wellness and look at why we're lapping it up in our search for so-called balance, let's quickly regroup on how we arrived here.

Wellness isn't new. It's ancient. Like, 3000 BC or thereabouts ancient if you take into account the likes of India's Ayurvedic medicine, traditional Chinese medicine and Greek medicine, and when they were first practised. The *Oxford English Dictionary* reckons the actual word dates back to the 1650s when 'wellness' was used to describe the 'state of being well or in good health'. In the late 1700s, homeopathy sprang up, then 100 years later chiropractic. In the 1900s, naturopathy—which combined lifestyle, diet, herbs and massage to heal the body and stay well—took centre stage in Europe and then beyond.

But wellness, as we know it in today's lexicon, was first conceived in the 1950s. That's when the distinction was made between good health (that is, not being sick) and aspiring to a higher level of functioning through health and total wellbeing— inside and out.

It happened in America, of course. A dude called Halbert L. Dunn, who was the chief of the US National Office of Vital Statistics at the time, wanted a new term to define how a human could function at their best, and he called it 'high-level wellness'. Seriously, who wouldn't want a hit of high-level wellness? In 1961, Dunn wrote a book by the same name and his buzzword was picked up by various health scholarly folk. The editor of the then top-selling US health magazine *Prevention*, whose former owner Rodale, Inc. also founded *Women's Health*, further championed the 'exciting field of wellness enhancement' through their publication.

> ◤ *The Rodales were the first to promote organic farming and living—I visited their iconic farm, and tasted its flavourful produce on my first work trip to the US in 2008. An inspiring family, really.*

Anyway, come the seventies, terms like 'self-care' and 'mind–body' connection were still seen as radical, cult-like in the pure meaning of the word, and definitely far from cool. Around this time, a few wellness centres promoting wellbeing as an inner journey of the self and as an alternative to traditional Western medicine opened. Mind you, they were seen as pretty flaky.

The next three decades spawned a bona fide movement—the spa and fitness industries grew, wellness high priestess Gwyneth Paltrow took up yoga, organic ranges made it into mainstream supermarkets and self-help experts under 25 years old surfaced. And then—boom!—circa 2010, wellness was officially mainstream and we all wanted a piece of this high-level good stuff.

What made wellness take off? We did. Women.

Basically, wellness was meant to fix everything. The promise was along these lines: if we paid attention to our wellness, we'd be able to have it all, without the stress, the mental load and the burnout. We'd feel renewed, inspired and enriched.

Women had plumbed the depths of mental dread, so we bought in. Big time. As American journalist and author Taffy Brodesser-Akner wrote in 2018 in *The New York Times Magazine*:

> The minute the phrase 'having it all' lost favor among women, wellness came in to pick up the pieces. It was a way to reorient ourselves—we were not in service to anyone else, and we were worthy subjects of our own care. It wasn't about achieving; it was about putting ourselves at the top of a list that we hadn't even previously been on. Wellness was maybe a result of too much having it all, too much pursuit, too many boxes that we'd seen our exhausted mothers fall into bed without checking off. Wellness arrived because it was gravely needed.

She sums it up beautifully, don't you think—wellness as a reorientation. Wellness helping us reclaim that much needed mental power—to be clearer of thought around our daily choices. Wellness empowering us to feel that we might just tick off the 57 things on our to-do list with a little more calm, ease and a little less *screw you* to our partners.

You see, as women, we are practical sorts. Despite our sometimes precarious emotional states, we plough on through our chaos, seek healing, unfurl silver linings and welcome things that remind us that life is more than packing and unpacking the dishwasher. Translated into wellness activity, we experiment with essential oils in the hope that they will ease our anxiety, we fast for a full-body cleanse, and drink liquorice tea to support our adrenals.

The irony is that we are more health conscious than ever—our search for meaning, connection and spirituality is at an all-time high. We have phenomenal options to optimise our wellbeing, more than ever before, but it now seems that this is, in fact, amplifying our mental chaos.

I can't help thinking that it happened when wellness became a commodity—something to sell. Wellness lost its integrity somewhere along the line and we were probably too tired to notice.

> 'When you reach peak wellness it's a whole-body experience. It's peace of body, mind and soul. It feels incredible.'—*Ange*

Your wellness is someone else's business

When we're mentally fried day in and day out, who doesn't want to buy into the promise of something that will make you feel amazing inside *and* out? I bloody do.

Some of us like our wellness with a side-serve of glowy skin, while others seek true mind–body alignment. Whatever your preference, wellness gives you permission to feel inspired, calm, mindful, confident, glowier, kind, limitless, enriched, joyful, healthier, nourished, mentally strong, pretty, thinner, muscular . . . in a nutshell: to escape. And, most importantly, wellness allows a more balanced life. Workplaces, and the travel, beauty, hospitality and real estate industries (you can now build a home that is infused with all things wellness—mattresses, air quality, the list is endless) and even car manufacturers want a piece of the health dollar. Western culture is wellness obsessed.

Wellness is a lifestyle.

Globally, the wellness industry is now worth US$4.5 trillion, according to the non-profit Global Wellness Institute. Yes, TRILLION. Now, US$828.2 billion of that is the 'physical activity economy', so stuff like sports and active recreation, fitness, mindful movement, equipment, apparel and footwear, and technology. Yes, today all this is packed under the wellness banner. For someone like me—and I'm guessing you—this wellness movement is insanely awesome and amazing. Clean eating, clean beauty, yoga apps, biohacking, fitness and yoga festivals and wellness weeks at work. When fashion designers and celebrities like Stella McCartney and Heidi Klum team up with traditional sports brands, it means you can now, kinda, afford their stuff. And, if not, H&M sells athleisure with a twenty buck price tag. You can have a celebrity PT booming through your headphones, you know exactly how much REM sleep you chalked up last night and you can track your fertility (in Silicon Valley femtech start-ups are raking in the funding). You can eat activated charcoal, drink kombucha, lather yourself in CBD oil and snort cacao powder (apparently it's the new party drug of choice in Germany). The word wellness appears in more than 30,000 book titles on Amazon. Heck, your pets can even meditate—true story, pet wellness is a thing. When you check into a hotel, the US yoga sensation Tara Stiles can take you through a chill-out sequence, you can meditate on a Virgin plane and if all that doesn't trigger your good vibes, try wellness travel.

I went on a wellness holiday to Las Vegas for an article a few years back. I didn't drop a single cent in a slot machine or drink any booze; instead, I skulled cold-pressed smoothies, did yoga in a mega-sized Ferris wheel overlooking the strip and sat cross-legged for an hour in a salt-rock cave inside the Venetian casino. I even slept in a 'wellness room' in the MGM Grand Hotel & Casino. The trip was bizarre and overblown, yet unforgettably fun. I returned to my crazy chaotic household much more zen—which only lasted a week, but still . . . There's also the truly woke wellness things that most of us won't do but will happily read about, like steaming the crap out of your vagina, forest bathing (actually, I do want to try this because why not?), and, one that Kendall Jenner swears by, the IV vitamin drip.

Wellness encompasses everything and it can cost *anything.* Who wouldn't buy into all this wellness shizzle (if they can afford it)? Women are eating it up—it's a fundamental part of our lives.

> ✒ *What's the difference between wellness and wellbeing, you ask? Well, not much and like me in this book, you probably flip between both and use them interchangeably. The dictionary meaning: 'wellbeing' is defined as the state of being happy, healthy and successful. Wellness is also the state of being healthy, while actively pursuing a goal.*

But there's a catch. Remember, the wellness industry is by no means driven by doctors or politicians; it is powered by businesses who want to make a buck. And while many of them do seek to make a difference to women's health and wellbeing, it's often tricky to sort out the shit from the legit, and to keep the charlatans accountable.

Even Dr Karl Kruszelnicki—Australia's most popular scientist, who has made a profession out of seeking answers to the inexplicable—has put wellness under his microscope. 'Every field of knowledge requires training and education,' he writes in *Vital Science*. 'And if a field deals with something as complicated as life itself, then you need a lot more knowledge. And this leads me to my big fat beef with "wellness"—that some of its "experts" have close to zero training or knowledge.' So how do wellness gurus get away with it? According to Dr Karl, it's all about tapping into 'the emotions' and 'the journey' and how good the guru is at peddling their stuff. It has nothing to do with science at all.

I keep coming back to Belle Gibson, she of 2014's hugely successful *The Whole Pantry* app and cookbook, who claimed she had treated herself for cancer through wellness and then sold that cure to hundreds of thousands of eager people. Except that she didn't ever have cancer. By 2015 she was exposed as a fraud, a 'cancer con artist'.

I was hoodwinked by Belle Gibson when I was editor of *Women's Health*, but I comfort myself with the fact that she also fooled big global brands like Apple and Penguin Random House. Belle Gibson was an extraordinary salesperson—a modern, feminine, empowered snake oil saleswoman extraordinaire. For a long time, no one dared challenge her because I guess we all wanted to believe her story.

> 'Wellness is half mental, half physical—treating our bodies with respect and our minds, too. It's fuelling and moving your body

so it functions how you need it to. It's making the changes in
your life you need to make to feel better about yourself.'—*Ash*

Behold, we have feminist wellness

With the rise of #MeToo, we've witnessed an intriguing offshoot
of the wellness movement. Have you heard of feminist wellness?
Basically, it's a marrying of the two movements. The 2018 *Global
Wellness Trends Report* named 'feminist wellness' as one of the
top ten global trends that year. They predicted more women-only
workspaces, clubs and collectives, 'where women work, network,
empower each other, unwind and learn—with much wellness
on tap', the rise of femtech and, yes, travel aimed at women's
empowerment. You know, trips for emotional healing after, say,
a divorce or the loss of a loved one—these are called 'painmoons'.
The report predicted the industry would go beyond being just for
middle-class white people (um, yes!). Of course, this all taps into
the mammoth growth of women's spending power: in terms of the
global economy, the future really is female. And the future is wellness, too, or so it seems . . . especially if our mental health keeps
speedily declining.

But this feminist wellness is a good thing, right?

Not if it's a substitute for the basic fundamentals of looking
after your health and wellbeing. The irony is many of us lament
that we don't have time to see the doctor to get our skin checked,
a pap smear done or to see a dentist for our yearly check-up. All
of these being the basics of self-care. Yet, we have time to nip into
Lululemon, mix up a fandangled new juice and bomb our bath
with unicorn-coloured smelly shit.

The marrying of feminism and wellness is really just wellness sold under the guise of feminism—a fresh way to market

something, this time wrapped up in a pretty pink box with a white ribbon. Feminist activism is at its peak and what better way for some companies to make money than to sell right into that. Ingenious.

The host of the *Feminist Wellness* podcast, Victoria Albina, put it this way: 'With the commodification of self-care, wellness can leave us confused about what it truly means.' (Sidenote: I've found myself warming to Albina's podcast wisdom.) Yes, often cult wellness is just a simple bandaid solution to complex, deeper emotional woes.

In a way, it's served up to us to make us feel better about all the inequalities that still exist, to restore our perseverance in the fight and it's that timely escape that Taffy Brodesser-Akner hit on. This so-called feminist wellness is not the fix for our over-whelm, our fears or our struggles with perfectionism. In truth, it ignores the fundamentals of what we're all still feeling: we were promised equality, we're struggling to work it all out and we're still wondering where balance fits in.

Remember: our quest to be well is a good thing

Nutritionist and author Lola Berry is a wellspring of health and her sparkle is a daily injection of sunshine into my social feed. We first met in April 2011, in the back of a white Toyota Camry on a one-hour drive from Brisbane Airport to Ipswich. Somehow, two 60-minute car trips make the perfect circumstances for sharing your life thus far with a stranger. She was a nutritionist starting to make a name for herself in Melbourne, I was a magazine editor from Sydney angling for a scoop. We'd travelled north to partake in a healthy cooking class to celebrate the opening of the first Jamie's Ministry of Food kitchen in Australia. Not sure if you remember these, but Jamie Oliver opened the community kitchens throughout the UK with the aim of fighting obesity and teaching people the fundamentals of nutritious cooking, like what broccoli is, and how to cut carrots. (In case you were wondering, the Ipswich Centre still exists today and a later evaluation by Deakin University proved the celebrity chef's ten-week program did increase cooking confidence and veggie intake.)

As Lola and I cut carrots like pros for our chicken skewers, we connected over our mutual love of all things good health. I was drawn to her effervescent hippie vibe. I liked what she stood for nutrition-wise. She was trustworthy. We kept in touch and I launched one of her cookbooks (she now has ten!) in a tiny vegan restaurant in Marrickville, Sydney, a few years ago. As I've watched her empire grow—a smoothie and juice bar called Happy Place, her books, TV cooking appearances, yoga qualifications and now her latest venture, a brain booster coffee—I feel she's always lived true to her definition of wellness. As you can imagine, I've met and interviewed loads of experts and influencers in this space, but Lola has always stood out.

'When I first started on TV I was that hippie girl who would talk about natural remedies and old folk remedies,' she writes to me on email (we tried to chat about all this over a smoothie in Melbourne a number of times, but . . . #life). I can just imagine the eyerolls from those morning TV viewers. She reminds me that we should thank our lucky green stars that wellness is so tremendously accessible today. She's right. When you're lost in the overwhelm, it's an essential distraction and potential fix.

So, I ask Lola, why do women more than ever crave—and buy into—wellness?

'I believe it's because we want to feel good, not just physically but also mentally and emotionally. We now know that the gut is hugely linked to our nervous system, so if you eat good food and make your health a priority, there's a good chance you'll have more energy and feel mentally stronger, too. I also believe it's completely natural to want to nourish yourself and your loved ones.' True that. She's right, health optimisation—I like that word, don't you?—is a magic bullet for our stressed and weary souls. When we're lost in the minutiae of our daily grind and that feeling of 'I can't cope with this shit anymore', who doesn't long for better health, increased fitness, more energy, mental clarity and a top performing immune system (that is, lower risk of chronic disease)? Er, me!

> *The ancient Greek physician Hippocrates, often dubbed the father of clinical medicine, declared circa 300 BC that the key to good health and wellbeing is fresh air, nourishing food, exercise and sleep. It sounds pretty simple when you put it like that.*

Our obsession with wellness has paid off in some ways, others not so much (more on that in the next chapter). Australia has one of the highest life expectancies in the world: WHO says we're currently tracking at sixth in the world, thank you very much. We also have one of the lowest rates of smoking. (Alas, obesity is still up there—the Australian Bureau of Statistics' National Health Survey says that two-thirds of Australian adults are overweight or obese.) But if we go back to the Jean Hailes research I highlighted in Chapter One, we're the tribe who 'gets' the health and wellness lifestyle (rather than seeing health as a preventative measure from illness). It found 70 per cent of women said they did two hours of exercise per week, and more than half of those between 18 and 35 years old reported they were in 'excellent or very good overall health'. Nice. So if we, as women, now report that we're healthier than ever in our bodies, I want to know what the hell is going on in our minds? Why are the stats showing our mental wellbeing is suffering?

So, here is the truth: wellness is seen as the modern-day panacea to our mental exhaustion. It takes you away from work stress, the relentless pace of society, your mental load, the second shift and every other thought swirling around in that head of yours. We buy into it in droves in an attempt to boost our flagging wellbeing—to find our purpose, meaning, connection and fun. And if you've got kids, it helps us reclaim some of that 'self' that was lost the first time we pushed a baby out. Boy, this is me!

But. And this is a big but. Within all this goodness, this promise of enhanced wellbeing—of a balanced life—there's a disconnect. Our bodies are firing on one level, but what the hell is going on with our mental health? Is wellness actually stuffing up our wellbeing? All this supposed goodness we're sold on social, by our mates, community and beyond—is it distorting what living a balanced life really means? If we are consuming wellness in such high numbers, then why are we still so overwhelmed, stressed, anxious and fatigued?

Somewhere along the way, something has gone seriously skewiff. I think back to Lola, who personifies health and wellbeing. She reminds me that a quest to be well is a good thing, and perhaps it's more about getting the balance right amid all of the marketing and sales pitching.

WISDOM
MEGAN GALE

Quick bio: Best known as a model, brand ambassador, businesswoman and actress. Starred in a few movies, hosted TV shows. At 44, runs her own business—lifestyle brand, Mindful Life. Mum to River and Rosie. Partner to Shaun.

Interview need-to-know: We meet in her Sydney hotel room among her bags, breakfast and Shaun's workout gear . . . which made me feel at home, really.

Q: What do you think: is balance B.S.?

A: Balance is a tricky one . . . I'm a big believer that balance is key.
      If I'm working more than I'm having fun, I'm not in a good place.
      Balance doesn't equal perfection, balance equals harmony.
      People think balance is doing it all and having it all, but I find that
      creates imbalance because you're wearing yourself down to
      create this perfect picture.

Q: The pace of life can definitely wear you down . . .

A: Chasing your tail, mouse on the wheel—a relentless grind, but
      we're doing it to ourselves. We need to give ourselves permission
      to pause. Will your world fall apart if you take a bit of time out?
      Probably not. But there is a fear that if I stop, everything will
      pile up and I'll be more stressed. But at the end of the day, at
      what cost to your health? There has been an uprising of women
      supporting women, we can do it all and be it all, strong, powerful,
      driven as men, the whole boss chick thing . . . and it's great and
      it's very inspiring, but also that's a lot of pressure we're putting on
      ourselves to do it all and have it all. Yes, it's aspirational but also
      stressful. Do it at your own pace—we have to keep reminding
      ourselves of that.

Q: I absolutely agree, well said. So, what gives you a sense of
      harmony?

A: It's 'me' time, time with my kids, work, time with my man and that
      usually translates into harmony for me. For others, it might be
      earning X amount a year, always having a cooked dinner on the
      table—it's different for different people. I don't think you can put it
      into a box and say, that's what balance is. And that is where I am

very big on mindfulness—checking in with yourself—because we can get so caught up with trying to achieve balance that we're not asking, how are we sitting with everything?

Q: How do you cope when you're experiencing overwhelm?

A: It comes back to checking in with yourself. I can almost pre-empt it now. I can look at my week and go, okay, Tuesday and Wednesday are pretty hectic, Thursday I'll start falling apart at the seams and maybe not be so nice to be around. So I will book into a yoga class and usually it's the best call I've ever made. I come home and I'm a far better mum and partner, and then more productive. But it's really important to do that without feeling guilty.

Q: It's so hard to lose that guilt sometimes, isn't it . . . especially in yoga?

A: You know when you're on the plane and they say fix your oxygen mask before you help small children? If you go down in a heap, be it physically or emotionally, you are no use.

Q: True that. You know what's refreshing to hear? The wheels fall off for you, too!

A: They do, the wheels fall off constantly. I'm honest on social media, but I can also be reluctant to communicate things because I will be misunderstood. I feel like sometimes people might think, you can't feel like that as you look like you've had a great life. Sure, I've had a great life, but that's not to say I don't have my moments. I'm very good at putting things into perspective, and I always remind myself there's someone worse off than me.

Q: You've had a real mental, spiritual shift in many ways. What's changed?

A: In the past I would've let things overwhelm me—when you have a job that's very public and you're open to criticism a lot of things are out of your control. I used to really struggle with trying to let go. My man has taught me how to deal with things without letting them overwhelm me—to control my controllables. He's a great person to have as a partner, as I turn to him and say, 'Help me, I am feeling really overwhelmed.'

'The wellness industry thrives due to a collection of complementary ideas, blended hard into a thick juice. One is the alluring mystique of nature, compared with the cold arrogance of Western medicine and its relentless evidence; wellness cures are rarely proven to fail because they can rarely be proven to work.'

Eva Wiseman, *The Guardian*

CHAPTER EIGHT

THE B.S.
OF IT ALL

I popped into a cool festival in Sydney's Centennial Park called Wanderlust in October 2019, where there were enough acai bowls to sink the *Titanic*. Sure, there was the mannequin-shaped crowd, but there were plenty of other tribes, too (all body shapes and sizes and ages). Actually, Lola Berry was there giving her expert nutrition talks to a committed crowd. While hundreds of women and, as usual, fewer men took part in the Mindful Triathlon (5-kay run, 75 minutes yoga and 25 minutes meditation), many snapping selfies along the way, others wound down with a 'sound bath'. (Translation: meditation where a gong hits a bowl and you are literally bathed in sound waves.)

There was hardly a spare blade of grass on which to flick out my mat for the class with Canadian Eoin Finn, a self-proclaimed—wait for it—blissologist. He took to the stage with an ear-to-ear grin, his self-confidence downright charming even from a distance. He had the audience hypnotised from his first pose, a yogi rock-star in every respect.

It was mid-downward dog when I had a mini-epiphany. I had fallen victim to the conundrum that is cult wellness. Being at that day-long festival gave me a solid chop-out from my frenetic weekend family life and I thoroughly enjoyed being with my wellness tribe. But no matter how well all this made me feel, I had still been drawn into the wellness *economy* underpinning the time out—businesses capitalising on my stress, selling me wellness cures backed by popular opinion and pseudoscience rather than Western medicine and actual science.

Let's face it, I was easy prey. Who's got time to filter through it all to make a fully informed decision about a proper wellbeing hit when it's so desperately needed?

As part of my job, I've tried many weird and wonderful things to boost my wellbeing. I made moon water for a story once. Yes, actually left a mason jar of tap water on my outdoor teak table to soak up the apparent good energy from the full moon. I'd spotted Victoria Beckham spruiking it as a health elixir on her Instagram stories. Hers was $80 a pop, you know, and came from some insanely picturesque, no doubt expensive, spa in Europe. Mine was free, probably filled with bits of possum shit and, honestly, it did squat for my wellbeing.

I also lived like a health goth for a week—dressed in black workout gear, slathered on dark lipstick and ate nothing but eggplants, grapes and blackberries. Then there was the time I did yoga for a month on a mat that resembled an ancient torture device. I think that one may have come courtesy of Gwyneth Paltrow. Sure, these were all road tested for stories in a bit of jest, but still . . . My point is, whatever your wellness bent, today there is something to cater to it and also much to confuse: go vegan, don't go vegan. Keto diet or paleo? Drink kombucha, but not with food. Coffee before or after a workout?

Because of my exposure to wellness trends—the good, the bad and the downright wacky—you would think I'd be hardened to the sales pitches for new cure-all products and programs. But because I'm overtired, lugging around my mental load, I still hope against hope there's an easy solution, a quick fix that will restore some much-needed balance to my life. I'm not *sick*, so seeing a doctor doesn't seem like the right answer. In fact, I'm *driven* to be well.

And this, my friends, is exactly what has elevated wellness to cult status—it's the fervour with which we pursue it as the solution. There are now so many of us like this and our dollar fuels this enormous industry.

In fact, we might have reached peak wellness—or at least saturation. I suspect the relentless quest for wellness is now doing some of us more harm than good. We're poorer for it, in every sense of the word.

Cult wellness and its crap

Whether you're submerged in a heinous work project, or your thoughts are monopolised by an alluring douchebag you met on Bumble you just can't shake, or a sea of vomity children . . . bring on the whole wellness shebang. Look, when I'm awake in the middle of the night juggling blue ice-cream buckets with beach towels and sleeping in different beds, knowing I have to front up to TV early the next morning . . . throw the wellness book at me. I'll try anything. It becomes a bit like the thought of Channing Tatum (if he's not your bag, insert your celebrity hall pass here) serving us pancakes with strawberries and whipped cream in his *Magic Mike* costume. Now, *that* would ease anyone's anxiety. Although I'd probably take Bradley Cooper over Channing . . .

Anyway, when you're swamped with life, the cult of wellness can be alluring. It offers hope.

Cult wellness—meaning wellness that has been commod-ified—can be a key measure of women's success and there's a subconscious competition that comes along with it, a healthier-than-thou attitude. Let's not forget that wellness is aimed at middle-class women and, in its commodified form, only really works if you have the money to pay for it (a true First World problem).

In my final years at *Women's Health,* after wellness had taken off, I spoke about all this many times in presentations to advertisers, many of whom were now decked out in P.E Nation. Research we'd conducted at the magazine proved that not only was health the new black, but that being 'well-thy' was the new social currency. By attending fitness festivals, sporting the latest Nike trainers and taking part in Friday night's disco yoga (that's yoga with everyone wearing earphones so the room is eerily silent) instead of downing drinks at the pub, you were part of the 'cool' health tribe. Of course, you needed it posted on social media for true validation. And if you didn't post it, your self-esteem might be ripped to shreds—or at least torn a little—and so the guilt cycle would begin. Well, that's what our research said. And yes, the advertising dollars rolled in, not just for our magazine but for many other media brands and individuals (especially via social media). It was like suddenly people understood what healthy, fit and well truly felt like and businesses could now make some money out of it.

In many ways, the pursuit of cult wellness is both self-absorbed and self-obsessed, with varying layers of narcissism woven in. It takes up valuable time putting on your healthy game face every day—time the majority of us know we don't have when we're overloaded with life, even if has practically become part of your DNA. I've witnessed this firsthand at, for example, the launch of a new wellness drink, where pretty women were more engrossed in their selfie game in front of the impressive flower wall than the supposed nutritional goodness infused in the product.

Many wellness products are marketed towards thin, young, toned and privileged white women. For the 99 per cent of us who aren't mannequin-shaped, who are in fact juggling mental loads, are tired and stressed and cannot afford to buy organic kale every day, this can make us feel pretty inadequate. Many experts have called out the wellness industry as being the diet industry in disguise—all lumped under the banner of self-care.

> ✈ *I just checked Instagram and #selfcare has been used 21.9 million times. One at the top featured Kermit the Frog drinking coffee. True story. I love Kermit as he makes me nostalgic for childhood but . . . wtf?*

The New York Times bestselling author Jessica Knoll wrote a compelling op-ed called 'Smash The Wellness Industry' that made headlines around the world. In it, she said:

I called this poisonous relationship between a body I was indoctrinated to hate and food I had been taught to fear 'wellness.' This was before I could recognise wellness culture for what it was—a dangerous con that seduces smart women with pseudoscientific claims of increasing energy, reducing inflammation, lowering the risk of cancer and healing skin, gut and fertility problems. But at its core, 'wellness' is about weight loss. It demonises calorically dense and delicious foods, preserving a vicious fallacy: Thin is healthy and healthy is thin.

She made some valid points, didn't she? Wellness with pseudoscientific claims can be harmful and damaging, playing straight into our vulnerabilities. It can be confusing when you're served up messages with trusty celebrity ambassadors leading the cause. And, yes, there are parts of the movement that are simply the new diet industry going under the guise of wellness. But there are other sides of it—like fitness classes, food and meditation apps, just to name a few—that are science-backed and expert-approved by Lola Berry-types. This is where I believe wellness is a good thing—when it inspires us to be healthier and mentally well human beings. As I've said before, it's about sifting the shit from the legit.

> ⤴   'When wellness became a hashtag on social media, prancing around looking good in a bikini with a green juice in tropical locations became synonymous with having a healthy life and so it became elitist. All the talk of juicing and clean eating and fasting has always been there, but it's a small aspect of the whole wellness picture.'—*Tara*

We're not doing wellness very well anymore

The way wellness is now, it can so quickly become just another thing on your to-do list—another box to tick that you want, need and have to have for a quick feel-good fix.

'The wellness message, however that gets transmitted to you, becomes yet another thing you feel you're not doing properly: "I've got to defrost the meat, finish that report, find balance, find wellness in my life",' Dr Rebecca Huntley tells me.

Oh yes, you must try that breakfast protein sprinkle shit, go gluten-free to heal your gut for a month or quit sugar, all while struggling to find a dinner option that night . . . and, my friend, we're drowning in the guilt of it all. The constant pressure to improve, feel and look physically amazing and serene—because we compare ourselves to everyone around us and those influencers who are paid to make it look easy—turns it all into a keeping-up-with-the-Joneses kind of thing.

Dr Nikki Stamp, the esteemed Sydney heart surgeon, health commentator and, might I add, proud feminist, wrote a compelling book that I devoured on a flight from Sydney to Melbourne. It's called *Pretty Unhealthy: Why our obsession with looking healthy is making us sick*. In the book, she talks about the moral judgement of 'healthism' and takes issue with the popular health advocates who fail to admit their flaws:

> Health is now advertised as a project, a need to be the most beautiful, glowing, energetic and best version of yourself, prefer-ably documented on social media in a carefully cultivated series of squares demonstrating your physical, emotional and moral superiority . . . a whole industry has grown in recent years that capitalises on our fear—a fear of being unhealthy—which so often masquerades as not being 'enough'. Not skinny enough, not popular enough and not attractive enough.

When I think back to when we launched *Women's Health*, our manifesto was built on the fundamentals of science-backed health. But the industry has evolved. Is it a good thing? In many ways, yes, because there is more exposure to the most excellent benefits of health and wellbeing. In other ways, no, as there is more confu-sion, scepticism and charlatans than ever before.

The Guardian's Eva Wiseman made an interesting point after seeing the reaction to Goop's Wellness Summit in London in July 2019 (Sidenote: fans found the $8650 price tag for the weekend

extortionist. Look, I'd probably go if it was $100). Under the
provocative title 'Is this the end of wellness?', Wiseman wrote:

> And there is a gendered claw, with a combination of feminist
> tropes—the idea that women's health is misunderstood and the
> medical establishment ignorant about our bodies—and a sly
> regifting of the diet industry, this time with detox plans and slim-
> ming drips. But for every new wellness fad—activated charcoal,
> pink salt, placenta smoothies—there is a noisy, science-based
> argument debunking it, and increased responsibility from trusted
> institutions who understand more care is required when repres-
> enting magical thinking and its premier philosophers.

The lesson I take out of all this, for you and me, is awareness—remind yourself that in your moments, days and weeks
of stress, at the peak of those destructive, sad thoughts, you're
ripe for being sold sheet masks and bath salts. You're ripe for
commercial exploitation when you're at your most vulnerable. Cult
wellness sells straight into your insecurities, offering you a quick
fix to your overwhelm, your stressors, your hang-ups, be they
balance, body or beyond. You buy in, get a quick hit of dopamine,
it makes you feel good, satisfied—even just for a moment. Then
you come back, spend more money and so on and so on.

> ➤ *Dopamine can be shifty, yet nifty, and the right balance is*
> *essential for mental wellbeing. It's one of the brain's four*
> *neurotransmitters that trigger feelings of pleasure and*
> *happiness. The other three are, of course, serotonin, oxytocin*
> *and endorphins. Research shows some natural dopamine*
> *triggers are exercise, eating protein, music and meditation.*

True wellness is actually the opposite of consumerism—it's a desire to be whole, connected, calm and complete just as you authentically are. This is the kind of wellness I love. Cult wellness, on the other hand, can stop us from living truly rich and meaningful lives.

You simply can't find an antidote to your overwhelm in a jar, drink or online program (well, not unless it's a good bottle of wine). Dr Libby is big on this. 'The health issues are not going to get better until women get to the heart of their stress,' she tells me. 'We think our stress comes from everything outside of us, the people, the tasks, the situations and when we see the stress as being everything outside us, we don't have the power to change that. We think that's how life is going to be now, whereas what we forget is it's our response to all this and it's very difficult to see that when you're caught up in the hectic chaos of the daily juggling act.'

It's much easier to 'add to cart' for an instant wellness hit.

Remember this: no one values your health as much as you do. They might place a value on your wellness spend, but your actual health—mental and physical—is a very different matter.

> 'The wellness boom is a double-edged sword. It's done good things—like brought mental health issues into our conversations—but I've seen and personally experienced the dark side, too. What's the point of going to F45 seven days a week and eating smoothie bowls at home if you haven't been on a date or seen a mate in a fortnight? If you're doing the 'body' wellness stuff, make sure you're doing the brain stuff, too.'—Ash

Wellness meets balance meets B.S.

So, where does balance fit into all this, you ask? Well, here's the link: we buy into wellness in an effort to regain balance—the perfect remedy to our overwhelm, or so we believe.

I've been trying to think about what balance looks like, and all I can come up with is the most balanced celebrity I've ever met. I've interviewed and met plenty of stars in my career, like Ashton Kutcher (sweet), Heath Ledger (flirty), the Spice Girls (Mel B was the *best*) and Beyoncé (more on her later) to namedrop a few. None of them were what I would call 'balanced'. But Miranda Kerr was. Look, I know you might be rolling your eyes at this—I get that—but hear me out for the point of the story. As my old art director used to say, 'She's a bit fey, isn't she?'

There was something incredibly peaceful about the world-famous model, who was raised in the country town of Gunnedah in New South Wales and now spruiks wellness—she certainly had her spiritual shit together. In 2014, I had breakfast at her house in Sydney's Dover Heights, and we chatted about life while a private chef whipped up a yoghurt-heavy muesli that would make even Pete Evans ditch paleo. She was dressed in a floaty white-and-red flowered dress, and she was sweet and warm and her skin was so glowy that I went out and bought her entire beauty range the next day. I still buy her Balancing Rose Mist spray to this day.

I know what you're probably thinking. Of course, anyone can be chilled AF when they have enough money to sink on chefs, PTs, beauty therapists and nannies. I get that and it undoubtably does ease her mental load. However, there was this inner poise, a kindness and confidence, that seemed almost effortless. She was very in touch with what true wellbeing meant to her, and understood that finding balance is a subjective pursuit.

When I stuck the now 37-year-old on the cover of *Women's Health* a few years later, it was one of our bestselling issues ever. (Sidenote: Pink was a bestseller too, more on that later.) There's valid reason why David Jones invested so much money in her over the years. Miranda has talked about the fact that, yes, she struggles with the balance bit too. 'I think the perception of me can be, you know, confused,' she once said. 'But that's only because people only see that side of me when I'm at work, in front of the camera. So they don't see Miranda at home; they don't see behind the scenes. They see the glamour of it all but they don't see Miranda standing barefoot in a dirty old house.' While none of us are about to marry a billionaire tomorrow, move to the Bahamas and stick up a middle finger to our mental loads (#dreaming), the point of my humble Miranda brag is to prove that our quest to live a balanced life means something different to each of us—whether we can afford a PA or a PT, we're all muddling through whatever madness our choices have created. Yes, those choices are ones I'm eternally grateful to have, thanks to the hard work of my fore-sisters (thanks, Betty), as I'd much rather be struggling with how to balance all the choice, as opposed to not having any choices at all.

The whole work–life balance thing has had a resurrection in recent years (the term first sprung into the Zeitgeist circa 1980, then lost its sizzle early 2000s).

When I met Marian Baird at Sydney Uni that day, we discussed this. She felt it had re-entered our lingo due to the rise in the wellness movement. Women's increasing 'loads' had also amplified its relevance.

'Self-care time is the thing that women lose more than anything,' Marian told me. 'As they increase their work and maintain their domestic load, the thing that goes is their personal leisure time. Again, it's a societal and workplace trend to bring in wellness. I am a little cynical about that because if workplaces just gave people more time and a bit more support, and work wasn't so intensified, then we may not need the wellness. It infuriates me when I get an email saying "come to the wellness lunch" and I think, *I don't have any time.'*

After Marian mentioned the link between wellness and balance, I couldn't help but notice the number of press releases that hit my inbox over the next few days with the words 'work–life balance'—products offering an escape from the daily grind, a lightening of our 'doing it all' loads. This week alone, I've had offers to interview influencers on 'how to find the perfect work–life balance' in an attempt to sell a fancy new gut supplement. Plus a posh resort chain offering 'parent, child balance retreats'—now, try to decipher what that would involve!

I also believe it's why we, as women, keep coming back to the whole 'having it all, but still wanting more' mindset. The one thing that we always long for, the thing up the top of our to-do list—balance—is the one thing we will never achieve. Every person I've interviewed for this book, every girlfriend I've spoken to, every celebrity (except Miranda, of course) I've chatted to, every study I've read—you get my drift—all agreed . . .

Balance is B.S.

Nothing is ever balanced. It's a myth that leads us to believe that if we do everything right, we will be fulfilled, live a life of true meaning, a life that really matters. Life will be perfect. In reality, this equilibrium is never, *ever* possible to achieve. You're stuck in a self-talk loop of: *I need to exercise, I need to be the perfect partner, I need to thread macaroni necklaces for my kids, I need to start my side hustle, I need to activate my almonds* (can someone tell me how you actually do that?).

'As soon as you say work–life balance, you're out of balance,' says Jane Caro. Dr Rebecca Huntley laughs when I ask for her take. 'Balance is a mirage without *really* dramatic economic and social change—the constant demand to balance things just becomes another thing on the list for you to do that you don't feel you're doing well.'

We walk around huffing and puffing, we *wish* we were balanced yet we're seeking the trendiest wellness cure. Have you stopped to think about the fact that your desire to be balanced might be highly destructive to your mental wellbeing? If you're always looking for balance, you'll end up exhausted—your well-being depleted. Oprah Winfrey once said, 'I've learned that you can't have everything and do everything at the same time.'

Maybe you've redefined 'balance' in favour of flow, harmony, synergy, blend. Arianna Huffington calls it 'healthy work–life integration', an approach focused on preserving your health and wellbeing and recognising that there is no secret formula to 'having it all'. My old boss at *Cosmopolitan*, Sarah Wilson, is fond of 'tilting'. In her book *First, We Make The Beast Beautiful*, she writes: 'It's when you have so much to do and you could list it all out and try to prioritise. Or you could just sit in the everythingness and lean towards stuff as it arises that feels right.'

Roxy Jacenko says balance only exists between two things in her life: family and work. While chatting with the Sydney PR queen about this—she survived breast cancer while raising two kids with a husband in gaol for a year—I ask her: 'On the outside, you're the definition of "doing it all"—how do you define balance?' Her reply: 'I think you can have it all, but I don't think you can have balance. I have two healthy children, a husband, I have a beautiful home, a wonderful office I bought with the decor as

I want it. I have thriving businesses . . . what I don't have is the time to be sociable. To pop over to my friends' houses. That's the part I leave out. Do I mind that? No, but my friends are my family. I don't have any balance. It's bullshit. I'm happy with that.'

Whether it's integration, tilting, or embracing the imbalance and not caring about it one bit, perhaps it's ultimately about defining your own version of balance (or doing away with the term altogether); forgetting how other people look like they're doing it and being 100 per cent okay with your chosen way.

> ✓ 'You can't do it all—and no one expects you to—bar you. We're so obsessed with life hacks and becoming these productive, shiny examples of ourselves that oftentimes it ends up being the exact opposite.'—*Ash*

> ✓ 'The whole idea you can maintain balance is B.S. You might get it for a day, or if you're lucky a week, but then something tips and it's all out of whack again.'—*Tara*

For now, let's control our controllables

So, where does this leave us in our quest for genuine wellbeing . . . for balance, or whatever you want to call it?

I've had moments sifting through all the research and interviews for this book when I've felt punch-the-air empowered, on top of the feminist world and bloody grateful, yet others when I've been downright despondent. Don't worry, I've also had many moments of utter overwhelm, tears, sleepless nights and stomping around the house rage-cleaning. I've wrestled with major guilt around not spending enough quality time with my children as my mind is shifting through stats to include or trying to organise interviews while also doing a *PAW Patrol* puzzle. Or being mentally present with my husband or saying yes to catch-ups with friends. Oh, the irony.

For women like you and me, balance, however you define it, isn't going to be truly achieved until the structure of society, our workplaces, childcare options, technology, the mental load and the second shift have been moulded, changed and adapted. Then women will truly overcome their overwhelm. But it just can't happen until we live in a truly balanced society.

This makes me want to give a big shout-out to New Zealand. In May 2019, Jacinda Arden introduced the country's first well-being budget. While many commentators poked fun that she was polishing her crystals rather than running the country, there is merit to her mindset. Her Minister of Finance said at its unveiling: 'Wellbeing means people living lives of purpose, balance and meaning to them, and having the capabilities to do so.' In many ways, this is where it has to start—with our government making valuable policy change. Men, most often in positions of power, and women, who are more vocal about the problem, must work together to find solutions.

So, what can we do right here, right now—today—if society isn't changing as fast as we hoped? I'll tell you what we can do: we can keep talking. Out loud. Let's talk about how we were promised we could have it all, but it turns out that actually meant doing it all. Let's talk about how feminism gave us more power to have everything, but we've taken that everything to mean perfection. Let's talk about how we've bought into wellness as a solution to our overwhelm, but a chunk of that industry cares less about our health and more about our dollars. (While we build up our wellness, too often we fall down through having a competitive approach—I'm more 'well-thy' than you are.) Let's talk about how we've chased this aspirational wellness at the expense of good physical and mental health.

I get it, you want answers, too. Like, how can we lose some of our mental load to reclaim our mental wellbeing? How can we find more time for the fun stuff, to find our sense of self when we're lost in the chaos of work, kids, partners, friends and social media? How do we find the mental space for true soul-searching and reflection? How do we avoid becoming a human-*doing* and instead remain a human *being*? What can we do today to ease the load and make more sense of it all, to live a rich life? And what does wellness really mean—to you?

Well, I can help. I have some solutions, some answers—not all of them, but perhaps some that you've been searching for . . .

PART TWO

WHEN SOMETHING HAS TO GIVE

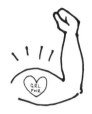

'We need to stop playing Privilege or Oppression Olympics because we'll never get anywhere until we find more effective ways of talking through difference. We should be able to say, "This is my truth," and have that truth stand without a hundred clamoring voices shouting, giving the impression that multiple truths cannot coexist.'

Roxane Gay, *Bad Feminist*

CHAPTER NINE

CLARITY: THE COUNTER- BALANCE

When you're lost in the unpredictability and uncontrollability of overwhelm—the household chaos, your mental clutter, body exhaustion, those crushing to-do lists, pesky thoughts of expectations, perfectionism and comparison, and I could go on—all you crave is clarity. If only you could add it to the shopping list.

I want to share with you the most poignant example of clarity I've experienced—a moment that's since steered so many of my life choices. I am sitting in my local library writing this and I can feel tears pricking into my eyes. Although, I can partially put that down to tiredness, mental load and this looming book deadline. Yes, right now I am mentally exhausted.

It was five years ago at 5.50 p.m. on Easter Saturday when, in our lounge room littered with toys, Tom and I had a frenzied conversation. I was cradling my second son, in his pale blue Bonds singlet and nappy. He was five weeks old then. I'd just taken his temperature for the eighth time in about twenty minutes and it had climbed quickly to 39 degrees. Really, the high temperature had come out of nowhere. We made a beeline for Sydney Children's Hospital.

The waiting room was swamped with sick kids. 'It's Easter; it's always busy,' the triage nurse quipped, but she immediately ushered us through the flapping plastic doors and into Emergency. By then, his temperature had hit 40.

The next few hours were a blur as doctors came and went, X-rays were taken, tests done, Panadol given and antibiotics were intravenously injected into his arm. Tom took our eldest home around midnight and our baby and I were transferred to the infectious disease ward. That night, still in gym clothes, I sat upright, hardly sleeping, clinging to him and never once putting him into the cot in the corner.

The next morning, with a temperature of 40 degrees being the new normal, we were moved to an isolation room with too many windows, which made me feel even more vulnerable. The doctors and nurses had to suit up when they came in, like we were living the movie *Contagion*. At 11 a.m., our baby was still limp and a ghastly shade of white, so the doctor ordered a lumbar puncture—a needle in his spine. At around 3 p.m., the results arrived. There was an extraordinarily high white blood cell count in his cerebrospinal fluid which indicated his tiny body was fighting severe infection, bacterial most likely, but it would be another 48 hours before the lab could confirm it.

All I was hearing was 'bacterial meningitis'. Yes, a bacterial brain infection.

'We don't know what we're dealing with yet,' our doctor said. Emily, that was her name. I will never forget her compassion, her composure. I couldn't help but blurt out, 'What about brain damage? Disabilities? Learning difficulties? Will he be able to walk? Um, will he die?'

'I can't answer that,' she replied.

I will always remember the hospital shower. The handheld shower nozzle that dribbled water like a beachside tap, the coloured speckles, like 100s & 1000s, circling the top of the cubicle. The showers were my lifeline, really—providing me with time to regather my thoughts, search for clarity to make sense of why this had happened to me, and an escape from the misery of that ward and the other parents pacing the halls.

When I was truly in the moment, I had one of those 'ah-ha' thoughts that I still live by to this day: my time with my children is precious—you just never know how long you've got.

It was Wednesday when we finally got confirmation of what he was fighting—meningococcal B and bacterial meningitis. It's rare to contract both diseases together, a double whammy, Emily told us—with no classic symptoms like the spreading purple rash. We stayed in hospital for ten or so days and returned home on my birthday, funnily enough. He'd got the all clear.

The sobering reality is that because we acted so fast, got to the hospital and got antibiotics into him so quickly, we saved his life.

After I returned to *Women's Health* following that year's maternity leave, the stress took hold of me quickly. Anxiety about budgets, covers and a shrinking magazine industry plagued my sleep at night. I valued my professional life, but I also knew I needed to be home more with my kids, not out at night at advertising launches. So, in 2016 I quit what had been my dream job and found a role that was more fitting for my situation: better hours, less pay and yes, new challenges. Sure, I missed my old job, but knowing what I valued meant the decision sat with me more easily. I walked through the doors of Sydney's News Corp office on 16 January 2017 to launch their new digital women's lifestyle brand, *whimn.*

It's time to do a rethink

There's a quote from American author and feminist activist Marianne Williamson that I keep coming back to while writing this book: 'You must learn a new way to think before you can master a new way to be.' If the fundamentals of society won't change as fast as the slogans on our pink merch would like them to, then we need to adapt, reshape and strengthen our mindset to cope, rather than just reaching for another wellness quick fix. Or wine. Or both. (Just sometimes.)

I know, I know, Williamson's weighty words are far easier read than done. As if you have time to master a newfangled thought process when you struggle to recall what you did last weekend. Well, I want you to take her words as something to begin with. Perhaps read them again. As I've said to you before, I don't have all the answers. I'm just like you, figuring all this life shizzle out. But every expert I've spoken to reassures me that we all have the internal gumption to get better at managing it, so that we can get our wellbeing flourishing. It's a matter of digging a little deeper. I have also unearthed some practical everyday strategies I'm going to share—some help-me-with-my-life tips, as a magazine editor I worked with once called them.

Tell me, what does clarity mean to you? For me, it's a lifting of the mental haze, a freeing of thought—I'm clear and I'm open-minded to face the day ahead like a boss. You know those moments in your life when you go, 'That's it, I know it.' How good are they? Clarity can be a sudden realisation or a deeper insight that you've mentally marinated for days, weeks or even years. Clarity brings the confidence to admit something you've always thought: that's what I stand for, that's what I am going to do, or say, or be. Or get rid of. It empowers you, it's uplifting and even inspiring sometimes. It's also reassuring. It has a terrific way of pulling you out of the negative and into the positive. You breathe deeper, stand taller, face life with grunt and power. It propels your mind forward, allows you to make quicker, sharper decisions. It enables you to act with your own sense of agency.

Finding clarity of thought when you're lost in the depths of boyfriend dramas, when you're burnt out at work and seeking the balanced life we've all been sold can be tough—impossible even. But it's the one—I'm calling it super-mind-power—that I keep coming back to that will pull you through those moments when you're feeling completely disempowered by your life's choices.

When things change inside you, they shift on the outside, too.

> 'Balance to me is clarity of mind, clarity of speech and an open heart (my yoga mantra). How does it feel for me? My body and mind are settled. Funny though, because it's not usually until I'm totally out of balance that I look back and see that I was balanced.'—*Lizie*

Be clear on the big life stuff aka know your truth

Your purpose is what lights you up, makes you come alive; it's your intentions or your 'why', as TED Talk celebrity Simon Sinek labelled it. Or what about this one: 'What I can do with my time that is important.' That's from bestselling US author and 'life enthusiast' Mark Manson—you know, the dude who wrote that not-giving-an-eff book. I like it, it's compelling. Mind you, the one term I gravitate to is 'know your truth', probably due to its feminist feels.

Actually, this know your truth/worth concept comes courtesy of the self-help queen herself, Oprah. I bought into her wisdom intermittently throughout my twenties, but then I witnessed the Oprah Winfrey extravaganza on the foreshore of the Sydney Opera House in December 2010, and I jumped 100 per cent on her spiritual bandwagon. Sitting a few rows from the front, I felt her energy and her charisma in full swing; I tell ya, she knows what she stands for and radiantly filters her life choices through it. I often listen to her podcasts now where she interviews philosophical thinkers and celebrities with a spiritual bent (they're instant inspiration for your bus journey to work, FYI). You have to hand it to the woman: in 25 seasons of *The Oprah Winfrey Show,* recording 4773 shows, she listened to thousands of people talk through their pain, dysfunction, overwhelm, joy and triumph, so she 100 per cent knows how humans tick—how they 'maintain hope for a brighter morning, even during our darkest night', as she put it.

Actually, she referenced the 'know your truth' bit in her 2018 Golden Globes speech, which was a rallying cry for the #MeToo movement and marginalised voices. 'What I know for sure is that speaking your truth is the most powerful tool we all have,' she said. Amen.

So, do you know your truth? What you stand for? Are you unequivocal on your values? What priorities *really* matter, like, right now? You know, often when we say, 'Ahh, but I don't have time' or 'I'm too busy', it really means 'I'm not clear on my priorities'. You're saying, 'My boundaries are wobbly and I wrestle with saying no.'

Being clear on your values and priorities empowers you to stand firm in your choices. This helps you shuffle those priorities with a bit more ease and guides your focus in the midst of your overwhelm. It can help you make sense of *your* stress with more ease. We see life through the prism of 'us'—our truth—our eyes. There isn't another human like you. No one has been through your morning, your day, your week, your year—those women lining up for coffee, they don't know the extraordinary mental energy it took you to get out of bed, get dressed and get out the front door. Or, the client in your work meeting—they have no idea you've just finished your fifth round of IVF and you're waiting . . . waiting to see the two faint blue lines. That rude Uber driver, she has no idea that you were awake until 2 a.m. finishing your university assignment and you're back at work already and it's barely 8 a.m. Only you know your truth.

I'm not a self-help guru (I'll leave that to Oprah, Mark and co), so I don't know the right way to peel back your layers and sort all this out. Or if there even is a right way. Apparently, some women draw circles, others use quadrants, write Post-it Notes or pick pieces of paper out of a baseball cap. Okay, maybe not that, but how randomly fun would it be to live by priorities lifted from a hat just for a year?

I only know what works for me. I write my list of truths in a journal probably once a year—the fundamentals are pretty much the same: family, marriage, work (career and finances), friends and health, but then others swing in and out and rise and fall on my list, depending on my life stage. Whatever brings me fulfilment, joy and meaning at that present time goes on the list. Not too many, mind you—you don't want to clutter your mind even more. In some ways, the fewer things on your list, the less stress and more living that happens. I revisit these truths often, too. And when I am deep in overwhelm, I flick open my journal (even if it's for five minutes at eleven o'clock at night after a hectic day) and remind myself that—yep, right now family is top of the list. That's just how it is. Accept it. Suck it up. Having kids was my choice. Career will be back on top later, and maybe even that volunteer work I've always been keen to do. I experience a mysterious centring of power when I read over my list. 'Remember when you wanted what you currently have.' I love that saying.

I reckon being clear on our purpose—and picking a sensible, safe number of priorities and sticking to it—helps reframe the whole idea of having it all and doing it all in our minds.

Sandra Sdraulig, owner of Through the Roof Executive Coaching for Women, put it this way, in an article in the *Sydney Morning Herald*: 'The alternative [to having it all] is to use our values to help us determine what pieces of "all" we want to make a priority and can honestly manage. At the same time to continue to advocate that these issues are issues that reside with the community, the workplace and the whole family especially men, not just with women.'

Piece together your values to create your own version of having it all. I like that approach. But more importantly, ask yourself what you can 'honestly manage'. If we asked ourselves this more often, I bet managing life would be easier. And perhaps you already do. Author, yoga teacher and mum Kate Kendall, who dishes up wisdom on her social media, put it to me like this: 'We're pulled in different directions with various masks, roles and responsibilities. We're never going to be in balance all the time. But we can practise leaning in to what matters most to us in times of "too much". Everything else is secondary.'

Quite simply, you can't *do* it all, so use your truths as a filter for your choices and stick to them. Be strong. I'm sure Barry Schwartz would agree with this approach (remember him—the paradox of choice guy?): his proposition that 'more is less' is ringing true. Loud and clear.

> 🎤 'I think you can "have it all". You just have to find what that term means to you. I'm still figuring out my own version of having it all. In terms of the checklist, sure I thought I'd have a few more things ticked off my bucket list by now, but then again, they wouldn't fit into my life today, and I'd never give this up.'—*Lizie*

Now, stand in your truth

The whole terrifying experience of our son's bacterial infection taught me that knowing your truth, what matters, is one thing. Standing in that truth is the next level of commitment.

I've always been clear that family, especially my kids, hovered up the top of my priority list, but standing in it meant being clear on my boundaries: saying no, pushing back, letting go of guilt, overcoming perfectionism, redefining expectations, losing the word 'sorry' and trusting my gut to step up. (I'll pick all these apart a little later, in Chapter Eleven.) When I resigned from my *Women's Health* job, I was standing in my truth.

I was chatting about this whole standing-in-your-truth mindset to a long-time work colleague, Tory Archbold, who owns the highly successful PR firm, Torstar. While Tory was at the height of her success, unbeknown to the rest of us, she was being stalked by her ex, the father of her teenage daughter. It went on for years. At the closure of her court case, she Marie Kondo'd her mental life. She told me: 'I learnt to get strong and resilient in my mindset rather than putting other people first, I had to put myself first. I stripped everything out of my life I didn't need—friends, family, clients— anything that wasn't aligned with my values or didn't have my best

interests at heart. I actioned my values. I gently closed the doors
on some relationships. I started pulling back on others. I was very
honest with people. It helped me stand in my truth.' It also freed up
her time. When she dropped this life bombshell, I was gobsmacked—
but also inspired by her resilience, courage and own personal power.

When you're clear on your truth, when you pay attention to
it—stand in it—you suddenly sit in the driver's seat of your own
life. It's like an emotional GPS, an inner guide. It loosens up
your daily mental struggle, lessens the blow of the little stuff—the
parking ticket, the 99 bits of Lego on the floor, the Centrelink
queue. It all somehow matters less and the stress becomes easier to
bear, because you're clear about what really matters. You empower
yourself to realise that you can't *be* everything to everyone, you
can't do everything—you only need to do what's important to
you right now. You streamline your choices, freeing up valuable
time. Only you know the path out of your overwhelm and that
path becomes clearer when you stand in your truth. That could be
pulling back on work a little, ditching after-school activities (do
they really need to do soccer, swimming *and* Kumon?), only using
social media on weekends (I dare you) or even challenging your
partner to organise *all* the food for the week. You trust yourself
enough to stand in whatever 'shit sandwich' (Mark Manson's
words, not mine) life throws at you.

I tell you, there's something mighty empowering about all
this. When you stand in your truth, you create a more well-
rounded reality. You think, you choose, you act—with clarity.
Remember, every thought, action and feeling—every choice—is
because *you* made it. As Buddha said, 'The mind is everything.
What you think you become.'

This is the most important part: you can become an agent of
change in your own life. How good does that sound? As Emilie

Aries, author of *Bossed Up*, wisely wrote in a recent blog post: 'When you're burnt out, you often no longer see yourself as an agent of change in your own life. It feels like all your efforts and your choices no longer impact your outcomes.' That's the crux of it, isn't it—when we are overwhelmed, we can't see the possibilities for change, let alone that we are capable of instigating that change in our own lives. So you default to blaming everyone and everything else and your wellbeing freefalls.

You are a product of your choices; there was a point where you made the choice that got you into the overwhelm. Only you can make a choice to get out of it, only you can tweak your situation. When you're about to throw the kitchen sink at your partner, coming back to your truth is key. Be your own agent of change. There's so much power in that.

> 'Speaking your truth is never ever as bad as you think it will be.'—*Stace*

Finding clarity of thought in your everyday

As you know by now, my husband was a professional athlete for eleven years. Sometimes I think I've taken for granted the wisdom he has imparted during our amazing (that's for you, Tom) ten married years—you can learn a lot of invaluable tips from elite athletes. It's nothing to do with how to kick a footy (although our kids also love this backyard wisdom).

Tom has made me acutely aware that how you navigate life—peppered with all its anxiety and stress—has a lot to do with your strength of mind and how you use your mental toolkit to pull you through. Funny, who would have thought the sporting field and bath/dinner/bedtime would be similar battlegrounds, but often that's exactly what they are. He cracks out this great line: 'Control your controllables'. This means freeing your thoughts from the things you can't control and focusing only on what you can control. I've found this sifting of controllables from uncontrollables a relatively easy mind habit to adopt, albeit without the rigour of a professional athlete. It can stop thoughts spiralling out of control and affecting the rest of your day. When I sat down with Megan Gale, she also talked about the significant impact her partner Shaun, also an ex-footballer, had on her refreshed mindset. There might just be something in this elite athlete stuff.

Which is why I found myself back at a football club while writing this book. Given that my husband is now the boss of the Sydney Swans, it's just plain weird to find myself sitting in the foyer of Richmond Tigers HQ, staring at the wall of shiny premiership trophies. It's even more bizarre when I walk through the yellow-and-black gym and brush past players who can't walk down a street in Melbourne without being mobbed for a selfie. (I always forget how imposing AFL players are when they're bunched together—it's their height and, er, muscles.)

So, what has overcoming your life overwhelm got to do with Dustin Martin kicking premiership-winning goals at the MCG? (If you don't know Dusty, he's that tattooed guy who won the Brownlow Medal in 2017. Dual premiership player.) Well, it turns out there's this woman, Emma Murray, who's been instrumental in the success of this football team; a high-performance mindset coach, if you like. And she's been kind enough to let me pick her brilliant brain.

Emma is not only an expert on the mechanics of your mind, she's also a pro at dealing with her own overwhelm. Her admission, not mine. Emma was a national under-21 netball player, and then went on to study psychotherapy and mindfulness, and now has more than twenty years' experience working with elite athletes and high-flying executives. She's an in-demand speaker. She's mum to four kids, and her fifteen-year-old son, Will, once a gifted athlete, is now a quadriplegic after he tragically broke his neck jumping off a pier in 2016.

Emma doesn't just speak about mindfulness in a way you and I can absolutely relate to, she truly lives it. Emma believes that the key to moving out of your daily overwhelm comes down to three things: awareness, acceptance and shifting. She works on 'how to shift so that you step into a mental and physical state that allows you to do better to feel better'. Bingo, that's what we want to hear.

Let's start with the awareness bit (we'll get to acceptance and shifting in chapters down the track). We're not talking about seeking more awareness from every other human, animal and cockroach in your household about the fact you've just knocked out five loads of washing by midday. No, it's about paying attention to what's happening right now (especially when you're feeling overwhelmed) to your surroundings, your thinking; to what you're feeling and your body's response. What's going on in that noggin of yours, moment by moment, day in and day out?

Emma explains that we need to accept that we're wired to focus on problems and uncontrollables—this is normal and doesn't make us bad, unworthy, flawed or mentally ill. The trick is to focus on your strengths and what you can bring to the moment. 'Once we reduce the fear,' she says, 'we feel safe enough to stop being hyper-vigilant to potential dangers. When we turn off the hypervigilance, only then will our mind allow us to shift out of overwhelm.'

Once you've reached that acceptance, you can change your perspective on the situation to be more useful and helpful, rather than being stuck in a state of overwhelm. Looking through an optimistic lens helps, as does simply shifting your physiology.

> ✒ *All the big-time spiritual blokes talk about being present in the moment. Eckhart Tolle calls it 'watching the thinker' in his bestseller* The Power of Now—*being attentive to what the voice in your head is actually telling you and calling yourself out for any pesky repetitive thought patterns. Deepak Chopra describes it as the space between every thought—a centre of awareness—and when you become familiar with it, it's your ticket to freedom from the incessant mental noise.*

Emma says most women have no idea how often we sit in a daily state of overwhelm, the nonstop confetti of noise. (She seems to know me and all my friends very well already.) The majority of us live in an unconscious world. The solution? Get conscious and call out your thoughts when you're trapped in the cycle, when you're lost in your own story. Now, by 'story', I mean that constructed narrative, your interpretation of a situation—like when you hear your email ping and it's one from your boss that says, 'Can you make a time to come chat to me?' Fast forward 24 hours and as far as you're concerned, you're fired. When, in fact, she only wants a rundown on one of your reports. Or, when you're fuming at your partner who's still out when they should be home to help with the six o'clock zoo. Where the hell is he? Or when you flick open social media and . . . FOMO. It's as easy as pie to construct a story as to why you weren't invited to a certain party or a girls' trip away.

We get lost in our stories, drunk on the emotions and the anxiety, worry, guilt and stress attached to them. These stories can be true or untrue, but remember, it's just *your* view. When you feed it with your focus, you can get stuck in that story, you can focus on what's missing, and it's hard to break free from the negativity. Your mind runs without thinking and the story looms larger and ultimately wreaks havoc on your wellbeing.

When you're trapped in an emotional storm, how *do* you find mindfulness in the moment? Emma shared with me the time her son Will had his horrific accident, when she could barely lift herself off the bathroom floor. Her story is harrowing. I fought back my own tears—seeing this amazing professional as a mother in pain is heartbreaking, it's real. I know that feeling well.

'He was in ICU in a coma and I was just . . .' Her voice trails off. 'I had been a regular meditator, but now mindfulness was an absolute lifeline. I needed it to breathe. To stand up. Do anything. I remember walking the halls of ICU and thinking, *Oh, so this is it—this is what it's like to be mindful.* Being aware pulls you out of the hurricane and into the centre—into the stillness of the hurricane. It becomes a survival tool rather than a wellbeing tool. It's not just about being present, it's actually finding a way to be engaged, when you're most challenged, showing up and doing the best that you possibly can.

'Trauma forces you to do it. Actually, I think it's a lot harder to do when you are trapped in a really bad storm as opposed to a hurricane. So, in our days we're saying "I'm just trapped in this noise of I want and hope and pray that my life will be different", but I'm stuck in everyday overwhelm. It's hard when I'm getting paid, I'm ticking the boxes at work, I'm ticking the boxes as a parent. I get dressed each day. That's when it is particularly tough to grab hold of your life and take it to another level.'

Noticing everything you're thinking and the words you tell yourself takes discipline; it's hard, tough. It takes diligence and practice. I'll share more on self-talk in Chapter Twelve.

Mindfulness, your way

You might be wondering why I keep saying 'awareness' rather than 'mindfulness', when it sounds like the same thing. Well, there's a method to my mindful madness here. I am asking you to look at the whole mindfulness concept in a slightly different way.

You see, I love the word mindfulness but in some cases it's shifting from the true Buddhist roots of the word (and practice), having been hijacked by woke wellness types and those who want to make money out of your overwhelm. As part of the rise in the commodification of wellness, the value of the meditation market globally already sits at more than $1 billion and is predicted to hit $2.08 billion by 2022, according to a leading US market research company. Yep, it's the next big thing to buy into. That makes me a little wary, and you should be too.

My other point: often when we hear the word 'mindfulness', we think, *Oh, that's too hard. I am too tired.* Or we think it will be boring and that we'll become restless when the phone buzzes and our attention span is challenged. We think, *But I live in an apartment, I need crystals, yoga mats and TIME. I am so unbalanced; I am so not mindful. Too bloody hard. It doesn't work.*

> ➤ Seriously, 'the average brain generates somewhere up to 60,000 thoughts per day, more than forty thoughts every minute,' write Jane Martino and James Tutton in their book Smiling Mind: Mindfulness made easy. So, cut yourself some slack.

And this is why I prefer to use the word 'awareness' rather than mindfulness—it seems lighter, more achievable and personal, and less commodified.

Don't get me wrong—there are many great people working in the mindfulness space. Smiling Mind, for example, is now considered to be one of the world's leaders in the use of meditation and mindfulness in the pre-emptive mental health space. I'm just asking you to be open-minded and discerning.

Because maybe, just maybe, a version of awareness, or mindfulness—call it what you will—is the key to finding a version of balance that might work for you.

The awareness that Emma Murray talks about is a way of mastering the moment—it doesn't require any more of your time. You don't need to attend a class. It just makes sense.

As I drive away from Richmond footy club, I'm starting to realise that balance can't be a permanent state. It only ever exists in the present moment. You don't achieve it in a tick-the-box way and then never have to worry about it again. It's having tools to fall back on that you can use to achieve a kind of balance in the moment time and time again, in different combinations and in a variety of ways. Tools that shoot down the overwhelm.

WISDOM
YUMI STYNES

Quick bio: Yumi has curated an outstanding career in TV, radio and podcasting. She's pumped out a couple of cookbooks and a great book for pre-teens, *Welcome To Your Period*. She can be heard at 3 p.m. on KIIS FM and hosts a most excellent ABC podcast, *Ladies, We Need To Talk*. She is mum to two teenagers and two toddlers. Her other loves, aside from her husband, that is, are working out and hot showers.

Interview need-to-know: We met for a 9 a.m. coffee. I shuffled from the school drop-off and shouted her a coffee at a bakery nearby (we live a few streets away from each other). Yumi is effortlessly cool, and after our chat, I realise she's a deep thinker . . .

Q: In one of your podcast eps, you have a super description of us, as women, being 'human octopuses', the full-time CEO of our family company—calling it profoundly unfair. I love this. So, how do you cope in this role?

A: I'm feeling pretty overwhelmed today. I've got to fly to Bendigo this afternoon to record a show. I've been to the gym already, made school lunches, I've got an ABC radio interview on the drive to work. My daughter possibly needs me to print her Year 12 drama essay because it's due today. So, I've got a lot of balls in the air.

Q: How are you juggling it all today?

A: Knowing the hierarchy of need—and knowing which ones can get necked quite brutally—that's how I deal with the daily overwhelm. It's about buying time, like getting takeaway. The best thing you can do is preparation, and experience teaches you how to prepare. Actually, this helps with impostor syndrome as well. If you're in a situation where you think, *I might fuck up, I might blow it*, be as prepared as you can be and then step up. In those situations, you've done your best. In the light and shade of the week, you can prepare for those times when you might be more under the pump.

Q: What about the ongoing life overwhelm—you've had some pretty epic media pile-ons. How do you let 'shit' go?

A: To be honest, ever since I was a little kid I haven't cared about the opinions of others. I do care about the opinions of my loved ones and people I admire and respect. But the opinion of a random . . . I don't care. People will always find something to criticise about another person. There are specific things I do in a pile-on: I don't look at Twitter, as it's a really easy way for people to access your eyeballs. It's a good discipline, actually. I don't know if I've always let things go—in each one there's been a lesson and until I was sure I understood the lesson, I'd ruminate. The first one was in 2012 and it was bad. I ruminated for a long time because I wasn't sure I understood it. How would I do it next time? How could I avoid it in future? Since then, I've realised you do come out the other side. It's a bit like when you've got a new baby.

Q: **It takes a strong person to speak up . . .**

A: Post-30, it's really easy to stand on the sideline with arms crossed, going, 'That is so stupid.' But it's more exciting being the one mucking in and trying, even if you fail.

Q: **When you were in that hurricane, how did you cope?**

A: It's surrounding yourself with the right people. My mum talks a lot about your soul. We're not religious, but she has this idea that you can be stained by bad behaviour and feel sullied and toxic, so I often refer to the idea that if you're doing good you feel good. If you're not being a good person, you leave a dark stain.

Q: **Your honesty is always something I've admired. I reckon we're not honest enough about the juggle and struggle that happens behind our closed front doors . . . and then we turn up with this Pinterest-looking pavlova.**

A: That's you, Felicity, not me. (*Laughs*)

Well, maybe.

A: A lot of honesty that's required is within ourselves. The world doesn't know about the state of my laundry, but it's actually bullshit that I have to do this while my partner is not expected to do this. In no way is he busier than I am at this particular point in our lives. That might change, but right now . . . I need to be honest with him, and if he doesn't step up on those fronts, that's him being a lazy bitch, and I actually won't stand for it. We need to enable him—or her—to do the tasks effectively. If you've got great shortcuts, share them but don't expect him to follow every single shortcut and do it your way each time.

Q: **It really does come down to empowering rather than enabling, doesn't it?**

A: The modern man understands that the reward from parenting comes from digging deep into those trenches—the mundaneness, the repetition—and showing up for your kids. Dads are doing more and more; my partner does school drop-offs and pick-ups which I find super-boring and time-consuming. It's in the daily grind that the deep bonds between parent and child are formed.

Q: **Do you think balance is B.S.?**

A: I had three years where I didn't have a job, and I thought when I finally get a job, I'm going to be grateful for what opportunity looks like. I learnt that lesson for three years, every morning. To work is a gift and a joy for me, and I will always bring my A game.

So, with balance, when I work, and I think every mum is similar, I work as quickly as I can so I can extract myself from that to go home and care for my family—my efficacy is watertight. The kids don't need me all the time, they don't need me to sit and watch TV with them, do home readers and a bunch of other shit that is fun to do, but not necessary for me to do. We do the cuddle stuff, I do the feeding as I express love through food, but I don't do the labour-intensive stuff.

Q: **So, you and I go to the same gym—how has that helped with your wellbeing?**

A: I'm there at 6 a.m. when my kids are still asleep. The gym helps my mental health—endorphins are the best drug in the world and there's no comedown. You go and worship at the altar of endorphins, hold up your cup and you're like, I've got them—it's good. There's no endgame, like I now need to get to 55 kilos. It's a spiritual practice—therapy—as it centres me and then eating really well feeds into that.

Q: **How do you create mental space?**

A: Once the kids are in bed, you know you've got some time. I have started reading again, fiction and nonfiction. I have a great relationship with my partner, so we hang and laugh. We don't really have the TV on unless we're watching it—it's never a background noise.

Q: What does living a meaningful life mean to you?

A: I really want to find this out, too. With climate change affecting
how we think about consumerism and wealth, we will re-evaluate
what being present looks like. Community building and helping
others in a selfless way is a practice we can all get better at.
A good check for me is to think about when I am dying—I won't lie
there thinking I wish I worked more . . .

'One thing I do for myself is—I holiday alone. I used to be a bit embarrassed about it because I thought it was a smug rich lady thing to do—and also that it could be interpreted as a rejection of my family. I have discovered that women from all backgrounds and incomes do it and it is utter nourishment for the soul!'

Yumi Stynes, TV and radio presenter

CHAPTER TEN

THE UNDENIABLE THRILL OF CREATING MENTAL SPACE

I've wrestled with whether to share how a trip to Thailand taught me the true value of creating mental space—whether it's for five minutes or five days. I suppose, if I'm honest, I don't want you to think, *Oh, it's alright for her, she can dump her kids and run overseas.*

Well, it wasn't like that. Remember a few chapters back, I told you how the #superwoman tag broke me and my exhausted, failing body coughed up psoriasis? It was then I knew I desperately needed a chop-out, some time to regroup, find myself—to sleep!— so that's how the trip came about. It was a long time dreaming, planning, saving and juggling act—I hadn't had a night away from my kids in almost two years. It was perfectly timed therapy. I didn't go alone—I dragged my sister, Eliza, along. We left our kids with their dads, mothers-in-law and carers, had list upon list of foods in the freezer, what-to-pack notes for lunches and reminders for library and sports days. As much as I wanted to just pack my bag and book an Uber, I cooked, packed and organised for the household to run as smoothly as possible while I was gone. We can't help ourselves, can we?

Finally, Eliza and I bundled ourselves onto a cheap flight to Koh Samui. At Kamalaya, the place we stayed (you visit here for an inward holiday rather than an outward one, their GM told me on our arrival), I attended the 'Mindfulness in Everyday Life' talk by a delightful former monk, Rajesh Ramani. There were about fifteen of us, mostly women aged 25 to 60, hailing from America, Kuwait and India, just to name a few of the accents I overheard walking in. We kicked off our thongs at the door and plonked ourselves in beanbags on the wooden floor. Rajesh had a dignified salt-and-pepper beard, wore billowy white linen pants and a top, glasses, and a wedding ring. He later told us he was a child of the eighties, perhaps a little older than me. He was calm and wise and smiled with his eyes. Despite hailing from India, he had a solid grasp on the machinations of our modern Western lives and how to weave mindfulness into it. To me, he was the real deal. About ten minutes in, he said this: 'You just need to find a little bit of space.'

It hit me: finding space to be 100 per cent aware of your thoughts needs to be a non-negotiable to combat the chaos of our world, your world. To help you not only make sense of the day, but the future too—to see through the fog more clearly. Perhaps balance is just creating pockets of daily mental space, relishing the stillness of the moment . . . taking the time to fill your tank before mucking in again.

Create a little more space

I love the whole concept of finding space in your day. It only needs to be a small slice of time, five minutes, where you can sit in stillness. In silence. Just to be aware. No distractions at all. Check in on your wellbeing, process your feelings. Anyone can do this, whether you're stressed up to your eyeballs with work, kids or meeting your rental payments each week (remember my overwhelm is not your overwhelm and if we compare we can easily get stuck in the guilt cycle). Just as Virginia Woolf wrote in her feminist essay, *A Room of One's Own*. That was in 1929 and it still sticks.

We all need rooms of our own (with locks!) to allow us to think independently, no interruptions. You don't have to buy a ticket to Thailand (that's what I call a total mental reset); you can find that space standing in your kitchen waiting for the kettle to boil, in a coffee queue, in the car, in a meeting room five minutes before your workmates pile in. Don't think of it as hard or just another thing on your list. You can sit cross-legged on your couch, lie on the grass, do a yoga pose, or perch on a park bench—it's all about finding a few moments in your everyday to quiet your mind, to be aware. To be still. And, no, it doesn't mean just chilling watching TV. I mean, Emma Murray shared that she regularly does it in a public toilet cubicle. Gawd, I love her honesty.

Sure, you can partake in the whole meditation shebang, I see that as the equivalent of chocolate for your wellbeing—just delightful. For me, when I pull out my phone for a meditation app, I get overwhelmed trying to find the best among the 30, but perhaps that's just me ... Look, I get it's flippin' hard when you have kids, when you're relentlessly taking care of other people's needs. Actually, it's just as hard without.

I found this journal entry from when my third child was thirteen months old—a time when there wasn't much mindfulness happening in my house. It was a Sunday in March: 'Three kids means you have no headspace. To think. To just do nothing. I have kids all of the time, and then I go to work and I don't have space to freely think. Maybe in the car. I need more freedom of thought.

I like that term. You don't have that when you have kids at your ankles . . . and now my daughter is crying.' (There is something about a solo car or public transport ride that can be surprisingly cathartic, isn't there? That's if you remain mindful and focused.)

Actually, an old boss of mine used to sit in the car park at her kid's day care, where she would take five minutes, music and podcasts off, to regroup, to mentally offload her day before getting out. I tried this for a bit when I pulled up at home when I wasn't walking into the second shift of kids, and I was still seeking to be present in my marriage and friendships, in life outside work. I'd sit there, take a bunch of deep breaths and say, 'Let it go.' This was before *Frozen*-mania, of course. Back then, it had this peculiar way of reorienting me. Today, probably not so much.

> ◥ *Creating a mental or physical anchor helps centre awareness.*
> *The obvious one is your breathing. The not-for-profit*
> *organisation Smiling Mind has this great tip: use the word*
> *STOP—Stop, Take a few deep breaths, Observe and Proceed.*

No surprises that the research linking mindfulness, and mindfulness meditation, to better mental wellbeing is coming in thick and fast. Basically, it's a bloody lifesaver for both mind and body. Actually, I found myself down a big google hole when researching the best studies to include in this book for you—there are literally hundreds and thousands. I then stumbled on *The Harvard Gazette*, yep, the official news source from the bee's knees university of research, Harvard. In an article titled 'When Science Meets Mindfulness', their conclusion named mindfulness meditation as a cure for ailments as varying as 'irritable bowel syndrome, fibromyalgia, psoriasis, anxiety, depression, and post-traumatic stress disorder'. Or, in other words: it helps you cope.

When you find space, you have time to reflect, think and plan. You get perspective, the chance to re-examine how you're doing life. You can ponder your current coping mechanisms, your responses and all those other destructive stories you keep telling yourself. You have space to ask yourself questions—to dig a little deeper—and hear your true answer: what can I lose to lighten my load at home? What can I do to dial down the angst with my ex-partner when I hand over the kids to him this weekend? I'm still single—what's wrong with me? How do I stop benchmarking myself against my work wife? What do I really want to do all day? Why do I care so much about what people think about me as a mum? Do I really need to go vegan? What can I mentally do to increase my ability to cope? Why do I talk so negatively about my body when I look in the mirror? Why is my life so messy? Why do I always say yes when I really mean no? Why is my head chaotic? Who should I ask for help?

The other important layer to this awareness thing is that when you are mindful, you have the mental space to feel your feelings, to sit with them. Lean into the spiky ones. Why am I feeling this emotion? Do I need to feel this? How can I stop myself feeling like this next time? Am I caught up in a story?

Pay particular attention when you're in stress mode. 'Get a clear model of what it looks like, sounds like and feels like when you're in overwhelm,' says Emma (who I'm thinking of as my new mind coach). 'For you it might be passive, for someone else aggressive. Think about when you're in a work meeting—what does it look like when you feel anxious? Close your eyes and go back to a time when you were stressed at home. In your relationship. Get a really clear picture of what it feels like and sounds like for you when you are in overwhelm.' Once you're aware of it, the feelings, emotions and physiological changes that are happening, then next time you can see it coming and use your internal tools to stop it.

A little later, after I met with Emma, I waited at a sushi shop on Chapel Street for my salmon roll to be made. Instead of pulling out my phone for a mindless social scroll or to check my emails, I put into practice what Emma had said. I pulled my shoulders back, breathed deeply into my stomach and really thought about how I was feeling. A little tired and heavy in the brain perhaps, but overall satisfied and content in my day.

A little space created. Awareness. Easy.

> 'I get up at 5 a.m. most weekday mornings so I can work out, drink a coffee and shower in peace. A little breathing space slotted into each day is more realistic for me than a spa weekend.'—*Tara*

> 'I'm hyper aware of getting trapped in the cycle of a busy life and have trained myself to take stock when I'm feeling overwhelmed and wind the pace back a bit.'—*Ash*

Disconnect to reconnect

Anne Lamott, writer, political activist and public speaker, says 'almost everything will work again if you unplug it for a few minutes, including you.' How absolutely true.

Sure, this can be metaphorically applied to any aspect of your life, but it works for me literally, too. Creating space involves one massive discipline that a lot of us struggle with: stepping away from technology. I sure do. Switching off and restarting for a clearer headspace is another way to put it. 'Sorry I'm late, I sat on my bed for 43 minutes staring at my phone.' Read that meme? Seriously, how true.

When Eliza and I were in Thailand, there were signs everywhere—stuck permanently and painted the same teak colour as the dining tables, for example—asking you to refrain from pulling out your phone for messaging, making calls or reading as a matter of respect for your fellow guests. That didn't stop people, though. And other persuasive mantras adorned the walls, such as: 'All addictions including socially acceptable ones can be a distraction to avoid being with ourselves.'

It was tough, but I held to their advice. When I was eating lunch solo near the beach, the rain dribbling down the thatched roof, I was forced to sit with myself, in silence, aware of my surroundings. I noticed the teeny pink flowers directly in front of me, a speedboat racing across the water, the majestic view. I was absolutely in the moment, it felt phenomenal. Technology takes us away from just being. From finding the joy, beauty and appreciation—to be and feel fully alive. Our phones, my friend, are contributing in a *big* way to our overwhelm. To our angst. They create a fog in our thinking and bring a manic intensity to our day that, really, none of us need. But we need our phones to remain connected, so the only thing to do is to use your time wisely.

When I worked at *Women's Health,* I had a peachy habit I practised every day. When I came through the door at night, I left my phone in my bag. I didn't touch it until the kids were dreaming in their beds and the house was looking a little more respectable. Then I pulled it out. Most of the time, no one had called. I seriously need to start doing that again—it's dead easy.

We're pretty lousy at safeguarding our own time, especially when we're at the mercy of emails, Facebook and the like. It's too tempting to 'just check' when you're supposed to be switching off.

Or perhaps that's just my rubber arm. In fact, this can apply to anything—parents, partners, kids, bosses or pets—anyone crossing the boundary when you're trying to partake in some silence, a little space.

Marie Forleo, American motivational everything (aka life coach, author, speaker), puts it like this: 'The point here is to challenge your assumptions of what you have to do and get insanely, brutally honest about what you truly want to devote your life and time to. Because, like it or not, your clock is ticking. Time is not a renewable resource and the only person responsible for deciding how to invest it is you.'

Fist pump.

> 'I find social media really motivating, but I am not always on it. Some days it's a good two hours and others, ten minutes. My life isn't on a screen, my life is in front of me, and one thing I can do well is detach. You MUST detach.'—*Stace*

> 'For me, if it's 5 p.m. and I've done my work for the day, I shut down my computer, walk out the door and go and enjoy my life. What's the point of hustling until 7.30 p.m. just so you can say you did?'—*Ash*

Running away from home

Alison Hill and I find each other amid people jostling through the Strand Arcade in Sydney. We share a small table and drink our coffee as other people's bags bump our shoulders. I've always been drawn to Ali's energy: she has an effortless calm about her, but that's what you'd hope for in a psychologist, I suppose. She's also an author, runs a business called Pragmatic Thinking and calls herself 'influencer of women of influence'. I like that. She knows her truth and stands in it.

We first met a couple of years ago when I was a guest on her podcast series *Stand Out Life,* and I've hit her up for life advice ever since. She's just returned from her own 'checking-out' break and I am very keen to hear details. If an expert does it, then it gives the rest of us permission to be selfish, to nurture our own mental health, doesn't it?

'I had six weeks off work,' Ali tells me. 'While I had the opportunity to do this because of a good leadership team at work and an incredibly supportive husband, it was also something that I had to do as I was emotionally not coping with staying on the treadmill. The time off gave me the perspective I was struggling to find staying in amongst it all.' But here's the thing. The mum of two approached the break with a sharpened mindset, a distinct intention.

'One of the things I did was to step into this time off with purpose—with a clear focus on my health,' she explains. 'I made sure I ate well, moved every day, caught up with friends I hadn't seen for ages, swam in the ocean and prioritised sleep. Often when we're caught in overwhelm, our own health and self-care are the first things to go. Having moments where you step back from it all and reset is critical to managing our own sense of overwhelm because it allows our system and our bodies to recharge, it allows our minds to get out of the weeds and see things in perspective, and ensures that we have the energy that we need in order to give the best of ourselves to those around us.'

Quite frankly, hearing that makes me feel a whole less guilty about buggering off to Thailand.

Coincidentally, I run into Yumi Stynes at the gym a few weeks after meeting with Ali, the first time we've actually done a class together. She's about to fly to Japan—solo—for a mental break and to write a new book. She reminds me of an email she'd sent me a few hours after our chat. It said: 'Hey, one thing I forgot to mention that I do for myself is—I holiday alone. I used to be a bit embarrassed about it because I thought it was a smug rich lady thing to do—and also that it could be interpreted as a rejection of my family. I have discovered that women from all backgrounds and incomes do it and it is utter nourishment for the soul!'

You don't have to jet off overseas. A friend of mine just books a night in a hotel near her house every six or so months. A caravan park is another option—book a cabin with an awe-inspiring view. Or maybe go on a two-night solo road trip. If you're a mum, you may have heard it labelled a 'mumcation', which I find a bit patronising, but anyway.

Writer Nelly Thomas wrote a noteworthy piece for the ABC about this. She lamented that despite decades of feminism, 'mothering is still equated with sacrifice', so when she was in dire need of a break, she decided to buck the stereotype and booked a trip to Bali for five days by herself. Her main takeaway: 'Personal autonomy is what makes us fully human. Doing what you want, with no consideration for others, is good for you. As the days of reading, eating, drinking and being totally alone passed, I began to feel like me again. I remembered how much I like myself. I needed that—I worked hard to be who I am.'

Whether it be six hours, six days or six weeks, having time by yourself—focused on yourself—as opposed to those small pockets of mindfulness you are now doing each day (you are, right?) breaks you out of your stress cycle and challenges you to sit in your awareness. Yes, to stop thinking about what the hell is going on back at home. Or work. Everyone will be *fine*. Travelling solo empowers you. You have the mental space to question your thoughts and do things on your own terms. It allows you to map out your future. To reorient yourself and remind yourself of what brings you happiness and joy. Sure, if you have kids or if you've left a partner at home, you will worry, miss them, you might cry and think, *Why the hell am I spending money on this?* But there's just no denying that a hotel room, wine and room service is a bloody good way to relax, recharge and rejuvenate . . . even if your family meets you for breakfast the next morning.

Let's not forget the fundamentals of good health

To be honest, it would be a bit weird of me to write a book about mental wellbeing and not highlight the importance of maintaining good physical health. To me, this is the backbone to living well. It also allows you to use exercise, food and other unwinding activities to create that much-needed mental space and, in some cases, get a hit of endorphins to boot.

If you need any further proof, check out Blue Zones—it's even been trademarked—which are places home to some of the world's oldest people. There are pockets of these communities in parts of Sardinia, Greece and Japan, just to name a few, where people live long, healthy lives free from chronic disease. Overall their daily lifestyle choices include a wholefood plant-heavy diet, regular moderate exercise, de-stressing activities (for example, yoga, meditation and prayer), and they maintain strong social support to give their lives meaning and purpose. Now, *that* sounds like balance in every sense of the word.

You might think, yeah, we already know all this, but you're too tired, can't be bothered and it's just another thing to remember to do. I get that. But how good is a little reminder? So here it is. Emma Murray said it to me. Lola Berry, too. And Dr Ginni.

Never underestimate the importance of exercise, sleep and nutritious food in maintaining your mental health, especially when your life is spiralling into chaos.

Often when we're as stressed as Trump in an impeachment inquiry (actually, was he stressed? Now I'm not so sure), or physically exhausted or mentally fried, exercise is the first thing we drop from our list. It absolutely shouldn't be. In fact, if you're going to make space for anything, make it movement. Emma has a lovely way of putting it: 'Motion changes emotion.' Isn't that wonderfully simple? 'When we shift our physical state we change the way we feel, which changes the way we think and what actions we take,' she says.

Exercise is a scientifically backed mood booster—not only does it kick off those feel-good chemicals in your brain, like endorphins and serotonin, it also increases norepinephrine, the chemical we need to moderate our body's response to stress. In other words, it helps us 'practise dealing with stress' more effectively, says the American Psychological Association. Look, you don't have to smash it out at the gym like I am doing every morning right now as I am ploughing through writing the final few chapters of this book. Talk about stress (my deadline—argh!), overwhelm (mostly in a good way), plus doubt (what if I don't have enough advice to give?), fear (no one's going to buy it, people will spend money and think it's shit), guilt (for not being with my kids). Writing this book, I'm grappling with them all.

A simple walk—just getting your heart rate up—gives you mental space, renewed energy and a more positive outlook on it all. It empowers you, boosts your confidence in life. Ample studies show exercise can alleviate anxiety and depression. And for an extra hit of 'I am loving life right now', take it outdoors. 'Green exercise' is a nifty little term UK researchers coined when they proved that outdoor workouts—be they urban or rural—really do boost self-esteem further than indoor workouts. Importantly, working out (indoors or out) also enhances your sleep. Sleep! Oh dear sleep—how beautifully it fixes everything—physically, emotionally and creatively.

I asked Lola Berry to name the one wellness trend today she 100 per cent stands by to get you through. You know what she said? 'Eat real food.' I might leave that point right there, shall I?

Actually, I will mention one more thing Lola said to me. 'I personally have a therapist,' she said, 'and I think it's like going to the gym for your mind. Think about it; we eat good food to nourish, we move our bodies, but we often skip out on our emotional wellbeing.'

Lola's advice is on point. Seeking help is still stigmatised, sadly—many of us see it as the last resort when we're in crisis mode. Thanks to more of us talking openly about mental health, this is slowly changing, but we're not there yet. Speaking to a professional could be beneficial for all of us, especially when our overwhelm is spiralling out of control. Also, when we're on the go, too busy to stop, that hour with an impartial expert—someone to bounce our thoughts and feelings off—can be a useful time of reflection. It's the ultimate 'you' time, in many ways.

Funnily enough, throughout my twenties, Mum always used to say this old cliché to me, 'Fliss, you need to stop and smell the roses. You need to stoke your wellbeing.' What she was really telling me was to 'create space'—to stop trying to fill every minute with furious activity.

It's only now I appreciate that quote's full meaning. Thanks, Mum.

WISDOM
SALLY OBERMEDER

Quick bio: Host of Channel Seven's *The Daily Edition.*
CEO and co-founder of wellness website swiish.com. Mum
to Annabelle and Elyssa. Mid-forties. Battled breast cancer.
Authored cookbooks. Is often seen with a green smoothie.

Interview need-to-know: I've known this effervescent
woman for ten or so years. After a few chats in the
Sunrise make-up room, we finally confirmed a venue
(with a shared laugh): in our respective cars on the way
to our workplaces because . . . the juggle is real.

Q: It's so easy to fall into the trap of doing it all . . .

A: On one hand, we're so competent—we can do it—but then you
    almost set yourself up for a downfall. You take on too much and
    when you can't do it, you're like, what's wrong with me?

Q: You're right—we feel we can, we're capable, we want to help—
    but there's a tipping point.

A: Totally. It's so hard when you're the nurturer—of kids, employees,
    friends—people will take. That is the job of a child to take, and
    your role as a parent is to give, but no one stops you and says,
    'You're running on empty, what can I do for you?' It becomes your
    job to do it for yourself and that's bloody difficult.

Q: It sure is, and there's a lot stacked against us—not just our own
    self-talk but the structure of society, too.

A: It's easy to say, 'Oh, it's just a busy phase', but the risk is those
    phases turn into years and because you want to be a trooper and
    you don't want to let anyone down, you just keep going. It's hard
    and exhausting.

Q: Tell me about the cancer diagnosis.

A: At 41 weeks, I went to a routine appointment with my obstetrician
    and mentioned to him that I had a shooting pain in my right
    breast. His care saved my life. A week after giving birth to
    Annabelle, I was back at the hospital to start eight brutal months
    of chemotherapy and treatment.

Q: How has your approach to the daily juggle changed since
    fighting cancer?

A: My overall perspective is different. You're holding a brand new
    baby and someone says, 'You probably won't make it, you won't
    live to see this baby turn one.' I'd thought I would just get old and
    grey. I never imagined that the universe would offer me anything
    other than that, then suddenly I was like, *Shit, that was a fantasy,
    something I just told myself.* The cancer reframed *everything*. On
    one hand, I have immense gratitude for every day that I'm alive,
    but the flipside is there's an urgency about life to do as much
    as I can as quickly as I can, just in case I run out of time. I have
    to consciously check in with myself and pull back. Beforehand,
    I felt I had ages. Cancer was a wake-up call that truly made me
    appreciate how precious life is.

Q: Perhaps you understand the true value of time now.

A: I can never go back to the naivety or luxury of ignorance is bliss.

Q: How did you keep going through those dark moments?

A: It was so hard. I really let myself take all the love and care that
    was sent my way. At no point did I want to be sheltered away from
    the people I love. I valued therapy—I needed that space. Even
    though the people around me cared for me, I also feared for their
    wellbeing. The arm's length person there to hear my fears was a
    safe place for me.

Q: Sometimes I feel we undervalue therapy to help us through life ... I mean, we're not taught how to do life.

A: I also just let myself feel however I felt. If I was feeling strong, I rallied and kept going and when I crumbled, I crumbled. There's a danger in trying to be strong all the time—I went with the ebbs and flows. I also said to myself, *No one can do this but me.* It's like having people cheer you on on the footy field, but only you can play. I remember saying to myself, *Even if I don't make it, I know I did all I could.*

Q: Tell me about the health scare after you had Elyssa—to me this demonstrates how easy it is to get lost in the overwhelm again.

A: If you'd asked me if I'd ever let anything get in the way of my health again, I'd say—no way. I never thought I'd have a second child and I was desperate to make good what I felt I had lost with Annabelle. With Elyssa, as I didn't carry her, I wanted to make sure we bonded as best we could. I would not take help—Marcus was amazing—but I wanted to do *everything.* I did all the night shifts until I got to month five ... and then blood just poured out of my ear [Sal had an ear infection and a burst eardrum]. And then I crumbled. It was too much. In the end I was no good to anyone—that was a wake-up call.

Q: It's so easy to lose your way, isn't it?

A: In this quest to be the best—mum, employer, sister—sometimes we forget where the line is and the extra effort doesn't always show in the outcome. That old thing that good is better than perfect, there's a lot of merit in that.

Q: Funny, that's become one of my favourite sayings.

A: Good enough is plenty. Life is a marathon, not a sprint. My husband says to me, but you can't redline every day. And I'm like, but you've got to make the most out of life, to squeeze all the juice. Yeah, he says, but you'll fall over and you can't sustain it.

Q: You have an infectious positive energy, where does this come from?

A: My parents did a wonderful job raising me and my sister. I'm generally happy and positive—I had a normal middle-class upbringing but somewhere deep inside I have a lot of gratitude for what I have achieved. My parents are immigrants—Mum from France, Dad from Egypt—and they sacrificed a lot for us. Sometimes I feel I don't have the courage to do what they did.

Q: I'd disagree on that—look what you've done and what you've gone through.

A: I also take full ownership over the choices I make—when things get too much with the girls and I'm like, *Oh, this is full-on*, I won't let myself fall into being the victim. If the business is too much pressure, I know it doesn't have to be—that I can stay or go. You can't have it both ways. I carry the consequences of those choices. That helps me look at it more like a speed bump and then I find myself back at my level happy place. If you accept that's what you choose, you'll get your power back as opposed to it happening to you, like cancer. So, if you don't like your job, leave, but if you decide you're staying, that's your choice and you need to get on board with it.

Q: Sarah Stinson, your boss at Channel Seven, once said 'your best quality is also your worst quality'. I love her wisdom. Why did it stick with you?

A: When I heard it, I thought my best quality is I work hard but that's also a negative—am I a workaholic? What must that be like for Marcus to live with me? And my friends. It allows you to become very honest with yourself and make change. You even pick on yourself with the wrong flaws—like I'm too generous, but that means you have no boundaries. It's really powerful . . .

'For ten years I didn't have the courage to say no, I don't want to work with that person—I was too afraid I wasn't going to get the job. Or, no, I don't want to wear that because that's just not me. I bottled up those experiences until this record . . . that's the story I want to tell.'

Jessica Mauboy, on the release of her fifth album, *Hilda*

CHAPTER ELEVEN

WHEN COURAGE CAN CURE

Courage—it's a quality and a discipline that can help you push past guilt, worry, stress and overthinking. (There's a sweet comfort in knowing you could do that, don't you think?) First, let's check in on that helpful dictionary again. Merriam-Webster defines courage as 'mental or moral strength to venture, persevere, and withstand danger, fear, or difficulty'. And it's the Zeitgeist buzzword keeping bookshelves bulging, podcasts booming and speaker circuits ticking over.

This is where I would usually share a story about a time I was courageous, but it's hard because, well, very few of us like blowing our own trumpet.

Mental and moral strength: do I even have that? Can I withstand danger, fear or difficulty? Here's what it also means: stepping outside your safe zone. Okay, I've done that before. Deep breath.

Way back in 2010 when I was editor of *Women's Health*, it was a vastly different sporting landscape for women: racehorses got more TV airtime than women, AFLW didn't exist and Ash Barty was thirteen.

I knew I was in a position to rally my team to give female athletes more media coverage, but I wanted to do something that went beyond our magazine, like a campaign or maybe an annual awards ceremony to celebrate women's sporting achievements. *Women's Health* couldn't fund all that.

A kind guy named Phil, who was working for the AFL, had locked in a meeting at Parliament House between the former AFL CEO Andrew Demetriou and Julia Gillard, the prime minister at the time. Somehow—and I'm still not sure to this day how I swindled this one—I got to jump in after Phil's meeting and had ten minutes to pitch Julia my brainchild, the 'I Support Women In Sport' campaign. We needed more cash to stage the red-carpet awards extravaganza that was to be the jewel in the crown of the initiative. It took all the positive self-talk that exists within the walls of Parliament House to enable me to:

A.   Sit in the same room as the PM and try to woo her.
B.   Cope with five blokes and a TV camera watching me do A.
C.   Reassure myself that I deserved to be there, using up her valuable time.
D.   Articulate everything I needed to say in just ten minutes.
E.   Be confident, composed, intelligent, smart, funny, witty and poised, despite all the shit that was going on in my head.

Guess what? It worked and our team secured government funding and we won a slew of national and international awards to boot. The campaign is still in full swing today.

What I'm most proud of in this experience is that I stepped way out of my comfort zone on several different levels and that I knew there was a risk of failure (looking silly, not getting the support or the money) but that I had a crack anyway.

Courage is speaking up in a meeting, accepting feedback, having tough conversations, getting married, choosing not to have kids, having kids, living pay-to-pay, moving overseas, making it to the gym, admitting you were wrong, processing grief, standing in your truth, *really* listening, sharing your ideas, resisting blaming, quitting your job, leaving a destructive relationship, processing a break-up, asking for help when you're overwhelmed, talking to someone you perceive is more experienced/highly skilled/better-looking, simply saying hi, making a decision, saying no, letting go . . . and even simply showing up, just as you are.

These things take *everyday* courage, but there are a few pesky things that get in the way of us taking that step into the unknown on a daily basis.

Ditch your perfectionism armour

Just as we're sold wellness as the panacea to our overstuffed lives, we can easily fall into that damn trap of believing that perfection will give us a happy, balanced life. You know that's total B.S., right?

This is not entirely all our fault—cue a collective *phew*. This messaging is thanks to a few indiscriminate factors like the escalating pressures of modern life, our brain's wiring, social media pressure and the upbringings of millennials and (some) gen Xers. When we were kids, we were constantly told we, as individuals, could have and do anything we wanted. Sheesh, we could be the next PM or Kardashian or Malala Yousafzai or 'insert preference here'. We were somehow special, life would be sweet, bad stuff probably wouldn't happen to us. No need to worry, we wouldn't be judged or shamed. Heck, we were even given medals for coming last.

Remember, too, we're heavily influenced by the social norms of people around us—in fact, we define ourselves by them. Dr Rebecca Huntley has some dandy words about this: 'We need to define ourselves *not* by what other people are doing, but how we can fashion a life so that we feel both that we are doing what we *need* to do and what we *want* to do. Plus, you're confident that it's equal—so that one person hasn't got all the balls in the air and the other person is sitting there occasionally throwing one in the air.'

How many balls are you juggling right now? Actually, I call mine spinning plates. They're all impressively colourful, too, some spiral spectacularly high, others scarily low and—oh no—there goes another one smashing into a million pieces on the floor. You know what? When one of my plates does fall, it has an uncanny way of reminding me that it's okay, I can let go; I can spin one at my partner, another at my workmate, and the day will still roll on, imperfectly perfect, nonetheless.

The other thing mentally weighing us down is the 'perfectionism armour' we're subconsciously lugging around, and it's not a flattering accessory. Quick reality check: it's as normal as shopping at Zara. Brené Brown says perfectionism stops us from being seen as who we really are—she's spent twenty years studying courage, vulnerability, shame and empathy, she's a bestselling author and general wise woman. Here's what she had to say about the P-word in her book *Daring Greatly*: 'Perfectionism is a self-destructive and addictive belief system that fuels this primary thought: If I look perfect and do everything perfect, I can avoid or minimise the painful feelings of shame, judgement and blame.'

It's so easy to buy into this false belief. The perfect yoga pose, the perfect wedding dress, the perfect partner, the perfect selfie, the perfect job, the perfect career, the perfect body (and face), the perfect bank balance, the perfect house, the perfect way to eat . . . Argh! Too much. But the clincher: finding the perfect work–life balance. Well, you know what? That's all B.S. too.

As women, we are too hard on ourselves too much of the time. Brené again: 'For women, shame is: do it all, do it perfectly, and never let them see you sweat,' she wrote in *The Gifts of Imperfection*. Sounds more exhausting than running a marathon in the desert. Then again, life often is. (BTW: I have done a 10-kay in the desert and it crucified me.)

You are enough just as you are. Yes, cellulite, pimples, wrinkles and lots of bushy pubic hair—it's what makes you, you. Sure, it's healthy to strive to do your best, to nail achievements and to improve and grow—this moves you forward in life, inspires you to do better. To find a fulfilling job, to renovate your house and pick a fitting life partner. But when you're driven by those almighty feelings of shame, judgement or blame—rather than wanting to do your best in that moment—that's when you're setting yourself up for misery and an implosion of self-hate. Strive to be a 'good-enough-ist', as Brené reminds herself (she also identifies as a 'recovering perfectionist').

I love that, I might make it my new mantra. Thanks, Brené, you superstar.

The truth: life will never be perfect, with or without your overwhelm. It's peppered with dips and curves and twists, and the sooner you accept that there will be arduous moments and challenging times—and you *will* get through them—the better you'll be at maintaining wellbeing. When you accept this, it's quite liberating, actually, and surprisingly empowering too. In her compelling book *Any Ordinary Day* (worth a read if you haven't already), Leigh Sales writes: 'The things you think you wouldn't be able to survive, you probably can.' And she's talking about truly heartbreaking, heart-wrenching moments of pain.

My good friend Dana, who 'balances' a successful business with a husband, two kids and a household, always reminds me that we're hurtling towards the bottom of our 'U shape' of this imperfect life. This idea is based on a comprehensive study of life satisfaction. It analysed 1.3 million people from 51 countries and seven studies, and concluded that happiness over a lifetime follows the shape of a U, with high happiness in your teens and twenties, before you hit rock bottom around 50, after which you start to climb the upside of the U again. Lordy, I have just under ten years before it gets better. And then you rise to ultimate happiness again aged 90. Yes, my friend, life in your thirties and forties is statistically harder—something to keep in mind—but it does get better! Once you are A-okay with the fact that life is imperfect, the day-to-day stress loses its sting. *This too shall pass*, I often say to myself, and you know what? It does.

Remember, courage is the mental skill that can help you push past all the worry, stress and overthinking. We think of courage being big, somehow—it's what our firefighters have had in semitrailer-loads, as do those who have survived and those who have stepped up in a time of crisis.

But it's worth noting this. As American author Mary Anne Radmacher says, 'Courage doesn't always roar. Sometimes courage is the quiet voice at the end of the day saying, "I will try again tomorrow".'

Hell yes.

Done is better than perfect

Actually, there is definitely something to this whole 'good enough' approach that Brené talks about. Jamila Rizvi says her work philosophy is: 'Done is better than perfect.' Jamila is a social commentator, podcaster, journalist, the author of *Not Just Lucky* and *The Motherhood*, a mum and an all-round cool chick. She told Wil Anderson's *Wilosophy* podcast, 'It's very easy to hold out to try and achieve perfect to the point that you become constipated with your work. Then you actually don't achieve anything good. I would rather put something out in the world that is good and is done rather than waiting for perfection that I'll never achieve.' Seriously though, what an antidote to our daily internal struggle — not just in work, but in every area of our lives.

It's about calling yourself out when you start getting majorly self-critical about decorating your son's Pinterest-inspired birthday cake—who cares if the racing track looks more like a car crash, it's good enough just the way it is. That washing that your teen-ager folded, you know what? It's a bit messy, but it's *done*. Your undies might not be put in the drawer how you like, but it's *done*. The present for your sister's birthday—just tell her it will be a few weeks late. Distinguishing between a perfect job and what is good enough takes practice, and little reminders and check-ins to your-self along the way.

I dug out a story I wrote for *whimn*'s *Body+Soul* called 'How I learnt to break up with "perfection sickness"'. You might be interested in this bit:

> I have always been someone who is goal driven, ambitious, focused—aiming high to achieve notable things—but it really took my first son's arrival for me to realise that sometimes you don't have to strive for greatness in every nook of your life. A new baby threw chaos into my days, uprooted my goals and made me realise that being too self-focused—and the desire to do everything perfectly—is impossible and just plain stupid. Sometimes, good enough is enough and doing a task at 80 per cent still makes for a rewarding life. You're not going to lose your job over handing in a five-page report instead of a ten-page one and, really, who cares if you can't do a headstand in yoga. One of the drivers of perfec-tionism is our fear of failure—we want to do things well and if we

don't we are scared it will expose inner weaknesses. This in turn creates more stress which then manifests in mental health issues. And so the cycle goes . . .

Remember Marianne Williamson's wisdom? The same applies here: if you change your thinking, you can change your behaviour.

We need to get to a place where we like ourselves enough to stop fearing what other people think—to examine our expectations rather than focusing on other people's expectations of us. And, anyway, chances are they think our good enough is actually great.

Over time, becoming a good-enough-ist makes letting shit go easier. In her book *Fed Up*, one of Gemma Hartley's insights from her many interviews was this: 'The most common answer I get when talking to women who feel like they've reached a balance is this: you have to let go. The clean house, the perfect motherhood, the laundry, the mental lists, the worry—it all has to go.'

Sisters, *something* has to give. I know it's easier said than done . . . but try it, even just once. If something isn't working in your life, loosen your grip. Who can you delegate to? It doesn't matter if they don't do it as well as you would. In fact, does it even really need to be done?

The Chinese philosopher Lin Yutang once said: 'Besides the noble art of getting things done, there is a noble art of leaving things undone. The wisdom of life consists in the elimination of nonessentials.'

My tenth wedding anniversary was actually a timely lesson in all this. Normally, I would've pondered, researched, agonised and discussed at length the perfect way to mark the occasion. But, as I was, er, overwhelmed with writing this book, I thought to myself, *Let it go, it will be good, fun.* So, Tom stepped up with gusto and organised the hotel, a dinner and for my parents to babysit overnight. And, holy cow, it turned out to be all kinds of amazing. Why? I had no expectations, no worry, I was open-minded and the best bit: I didn't have to organise it.

To quote Sheryl Sandberg: 'Trying to do it all and expecting it all can be done exactly right is a recipe for disappointment. Perfection is the enemy.'

> 'I've been managing my overwhelm by just taking a deep breath and thinking "Judge away world, 60 per cent is good enough."'—*Lizie*

> 'I find it helpful to think of things in cycles and to speed up and use that get-shit-done energy when it's required, but to slow down and do the slow things you enjoy when there's a day or an afternoon for that.'—*Tara*

So, what do your emotional boundaries look like?

When Ali Hill and I caught up, I was keen to find out if there was a common theme that unified all of us who took part in the 84 episodes of her *Stand Out Life* podcast. 'Let me think about it,' she replied. The next week, she emailed me: 'The importance and struggle with setting boundaries around our time and energy. As women, we find it difficult to do, let alone talk about how important it is.'

She's right. Often when we say yes to an extra work project, when we're late *again* to pick up our child from day care, or we take a comment from a friend on social media personally, or fail to stand up for ourselves with our partner, it says our boundaries are skewiff. Setting boundaries around emotions and energy takes courage, practice, self-assurance and self-awareness. In many ways, I feel this is a life-long quest—but if we can try it, stake out those boundaries regularly, our wellbeing will thank us.

As Ali puts it in her book, *Stand Out:* 'In order to set boundaries that stick, we need to first have the courage to admit them to ourselves, and then the courage to speak them and the courage to back them.'

Yes to that.

When I interviewed Jane Caro, she shared this inspiring story of a woman she'd just met—around 45 years old with six kids, Muslim and living on the poverty line. She'd just started a drop-in community support centre with a supermarket attached in Sydney's West. You only needed a gold-coin donation to buy food. In Jane's words: 'She said this wonderful thing when I asked what drives her and it applies to all women. She said a lot of women have trouble seeing themselves as a whole entity. They see themselves in relation to everything else—their husband, parents, friends—so they're constantly trying to second-guess how other people are feeling and trying to control and fix those feelings. This is understandable as it's a survival tactic when you're the low status person, but it's also completely destructive. This drove her to a very dark place and she sought therapy, and she realised that she had to replenish herself before she could actually be good at giving to others.' That's Megan Gale's 'fit your own mask before others' learning right there, checking in with yourself first and then erecting and sticking to your boundaries—being clear on who you're going to 'give' to—or . . . burnout.

The nub of this is boundaries—women feel they have to give, give, give, which actually means our boundaries are translucent, limp or non-existent. Often we feel that if anyone is unhappy in our families or friendships, it's our responsibility to fix it. We have to learn where we stop and other people start. As the ancient philosopher Rumi said, 'Your task is not to seek for love, but merely to seek and find all the barriers within yourself that you have built against it.'

> ⚑ *But how do you actually say no? Try one of these: 'Thank you for the offer, I can't right now.' Or, 'My diary is looking full.' This maybe: 'I'll have to pass this time.' What about 'That's not going to work for me.' Or a simple 'No, thank you' often works best.*

Your boundaries can pivot off your list of truths—knowing what you will and won't accept, where you draw the line, when to push back or not, and being consistent and realistic. They can be flexible, different for different people, fluid. 'The truth is we teach people how to treat us,' writes Ali. 'If something is frustrating you or leaving you feeling resentful, it's often because you haven't pulled it up or called it out. One of the reasons we don't stand behind the boundaries we want to set is because of the tyranny of "being liked".' (It's also one of the reasons we can't and don't say no.) Boundaries can be helpful in everyday little things, like when someone asks to meet you for lunch, but you barely have time to move from your desk. Say no, maybe a coffee in a few weeks . . . and don't feel guilty. Other times, like deciding not to respond to emails after hours or dial into meetings on your one day off, are about ditching the word 'sorry' and sticking to a 'no'. It means having the hard conversations even when you're absolutely fearful of the answer, like if your partner rolls in at ten o'clock every Friday night. Or gently letting go of a friend who's always asking for favours. Ali says the key is having the *courage* to set boundaries and the *conviction* to make them stick.

But try to ensure that you use your words with kindness, not as a weapon; be gentle, respectful and firm.

> 🔊 'To help regain a bit of balance in my life, I've set really clear boundaries when it comes to managing my time. When I started saying "no more" to things I couldn't fit in (or frankly didn't want to do), life started to feel a whole lot less overwhelming.'—*Ash*

Vulnerability, honesty . . . it helps

There's one celebrity who I believe defines what authentic honesty is: she's balanced in the vulnerability she shows and she is clear about who she is, from her inner strength to outer badass toughness. You guessed it. Pink. I first met her circa 2000, in a sunny photographic studio in Sydney's Surry Hills. It was the era of bubble gum pop and we had an hour or so to interview and shoot her for the next cover of *Girlfriend* magazine, my first job out of uni. I always got a little anxious before our A-list cover shoots back then, nervous that the celebrity would not be as friendly as they portrayed in their public life. I lost that nervousness over the years, or maybe I finally realised that fame is a farce—people are people at the end of the day and some celebrities are nice, others not. She was unapologetically relatable back then in calling out her body— worried about showing her (insanely flat) stomach for the cover.

The few times I've interviewed her since, not much has changed except she's a little more guarded. 'You can't please everyone. You just have to be able to get up in the morning and look at yourself in the mirror and like what you see,' she said. She's honest, vulnerable, raw and real. Pink's a role model we all need. I feel Carrie Bickmore's got this sorted, too. There's an authentic post on her social feed, where she's scrunching her fore-head, wrinkles on full display. The caption says:

> Evie: 'Mummy, what are those stripes on your forehead?'
> Carrie: 'They are wrinkles, honey.'
> Evie: 'Why don't I have them?'
> Carrie: ''Cause mummy is old.'

Quickly scrolling through the nearly 700 comments applauding her honesty, it makes me realise we need more of this in the world. Not wrinkles, just honesty. And in real life, not just on social.

When I chatted with Yumi Stynes, I lamented how we, as women roving the jungle of life, often aren't honest enough like this with each other. We lack time to fully unload, we are acutely aware that everyone is as stretched as we are, so we say yes to helping out at our friend's barbecue, we fall apart and still turn up with the pavlova (hint: next time, just grab one from Coles—they're good!). Or we're not honest enough about what a shit show, literally, parenting is. We all hold an ingrained fear of being judged which can stop us from airing our less-than-perfect parts.

> ✒ *Perhaps we're getting a bit better at this. Social media is shifting, slightly, and TV shows like the ABC's genius* The Letdown *sure help. This increase in honesty has made me realise that we all have our own version of what kind of 'mother' we'll be and, simply, you will not live up to that ideal. But you will be a good—no, a great—mother nonetheless.*

While researching courage and vulnerability as a remedy for our overwhelm, I came across Kemi Nekvapil, a speaker and author from Melbourne. I warmed to her as soon as I saw her energetic pictures online. Her Nigerian parents fostered her out to the UK so she could have an English education and she went on to try acting before getting into the raw food space. Fast forward and now she's an executive coach. She is also raising two teenagers. Her pitch is this: 'It's the really small shifts we make that make a difference, especially for women.' How good.

Spookily, the very next day I got an email from her PR promoting her successful podcast, *The Shift Series*. And when I met Ali, she mentioned how her friend Kemi had flown to Texas to do a three-and-a-half-day course with the guru herself, Brené Brown. Isn't it funny how life works like that? We needed to chat.

I'm keen for morning coffee in Melbourne with Kemi, but instead we catch up on the phone. I'm sitting on my hoodie (the grass is wet), on the banks of the Yarra River with my notes sprawled beside me like a nest. I wonder if saying no to a coffee is part of her boundary setting. I suddenly respect her more. She answers the phone with a British accent, although she's just officially become an Australian citizen.

'There is so much marketing geared at telling us that we're inherently wrong—our bodies, the pitch of our voices. You know what you need to do, not what the Instagram influencer tells you that you should be doing. The default is, I've failed and I'm wrong again. The idea for me is that we can all shift moment by moment in really small ways, meaningful ways—sometimes that's all we need.'

I ask her what vulnerability and honesty look like in her life.

'As the speaker, I'll stand up and I'll share what is going on with me—where I have struggled because I know that's what I connect with—it is giving ourselves permission to be seen.' Then, in her home life, she talks about how she's feeling her way around raising two teenagers. How just the other day she had a conversation with her fourteen-year-old. She said to her son, 'You know what? I've never done this before, I've never raised a fourteen-year-old. We are going to make mistakes. And what I request is that we're respectful in the way we speak to each other.'

Dr Libby has a thought-provoking way of figuring this all out, too. At her event, she asked us to name our 'forehead words'. In a nutshell, they are traits, or words, you scrawl in invisible texta on your forehead—descriptions that you hope to portray yourself as to others. This, in turn, depletes your health and wellbeing.

'It takes great courage working out your constructed identity as opposed to your real one,' she said. 'Wired into us is the fear that if we aren't seen by our forehead words, we risk losing love or respect, being liked or appreciated.' Fear wrapped up in expectations laid down by ourselves and others.

Dr Libby used two examples to help you work out your forehead words. When you're running late, what are you worried people will think of you? That they will think you're flaky or unreliable? And, if you're asked out to dinner with your friends but your body is screaming 'Nooooooo', should you actually go? It stresses you out saying no. Will they see you as selfish (something most women struggle with) or lacking integrity? Only you can answer that one.

There is a flip side to all this: it's called the big overshare. Emma Murray (my adopted mind coach) warned me that it's like some of us have been tripped up by the true meaning of Brené's vulnerability. 'Thinking you need to go to work and tell people that you were abused as a child or something like that. When being vulnerable is just saying, "I was really worried that I was going to do a bad job." We don't have to share our most traumatic experiences, it can just be the day to day. It's as simple as recognising: I am not perfect, and I don't have all the answers. It's okay to get it wrong, but at least you're having a crack.'

There's a difference between honesty and oversharing. Let's give Brené the final word. After all, she put vulnerability on the map with her 2010 TEDx Talk (viewed over 45 million times): 'Oversharing isn't vulnerability—they're not the same thing. Sharing about your bikini wax or the intimate details about your divorce isn't vulnerability. We need to be mindful and responsible about how we communicate with others.'

> ◢ 'I struggle with the vulnerability stuff in my online business. On one hand, I need to look like I have it all together, on the other I want to show the whole picture. I call my mum a lot and ask what she would do. I really value other people's life path.'—*Stace*

What courageous women have in common

I've come across some pretty courageous women in my life. My mum, a magnificently kind, giving and nurturing soul who sacrificed *a lot* to raise four kids and still does today for her grandkids (shout-out to my dad, too!). My sisters, who have featured throughout this book, and sister-in-law, Vanessa. After finishing her doctorate in epidemiology, Ness, along with my feminist-flag-flying brother, Bo, and my niece, moved to Monnetier-Mornex, France, where she now works at WHO in Geneva. Starting a new life with a one-year-old somewhere you don't speak the language is courageous. Not sure I could do that. My grandmother, who went blind in the final few decades of her life, and my other grandmother, who worked full-time in an era where it wasn't acceptable for women to work. There's the girlfriend who lost her seven-year-old son to a rare form of brain cancer one year from diagnosis. I mean, how do you crawl out of bed and care for your other two children after that? There's one of my best friends, Chloe, who lost her mum to breast cancer. Another who's high up in a multi-million-dollar business with a tonne of male reports.

Courageous women are my ultimate form of inspiration. Come to think of it, there's a bunch of others who've had a profound impact on me—our sportswomen—for their courage in the face of competition, setbacks and fighting for their voices to be heard. Throughout my years at *Women's Health*, I got to know a few of them. Freestyle skiing gold medallist Lydia Lassila, who at the 2014 Winter Olympics tried a quad-twisting triple somersault which if she landed would've made her the first woman to do so. She missed it and took home bronze. It takes courage to have a crack in the first place and then more courage to get back up. Track cyclist Anna Meares, who broke her neck in 2008, got back on her bike and competed in two more Olympics. AFLW player Daisy Pearce, who was backstage pumping breastmilk for her twins while hosting the 2019 AFL Brownlow Awards. Surfers Layne Beachley, Steph Gilmore and Sally Fitzgibbons . . . I could go on and on. But you know the one thing these strong, empowered women all have in common: an infectious optimism about life.

I prefer the word optimism over positivity—somehow that one's been ambushed by social media memes. Optimism is more a glass-half-full feeling, rather than a stack of hashtags, such as #blessed and #lovinglife. Harvesting optimism is a clever little trick to yank you out of a gloomy headspace—which can often be the one thing holding you back. I know, it's hard high-fiving your desk buddy on a stormy day—when you're time-poor and *tired*. Funny, when I am super tired I annoyingly procrastinate more (this is

a big one: replacing difficult tasks with something easier for a
quick-hit mood boost) which further fuels my overwhelm.

Not sure if you know this, but our brains have an inbuilt
negativity bias. Martin Seligman, the father of positive psychology,
has talked a lot about this over the years, including writing a
bestselling book called *Learned Optimism*, which focuses on how
to action optimism. Research shows that we're wired to focus on
the negative to better make sense of our world, we learn more and
it helps steer our future decisions—the negative stuff sticks in our
memories. It's why we can't help but click on the horrific Facebook
stories (and kick ourselves afterwards), why we ruminate over
our partner's flaws and remember only the constructive feedback
in our performance review. Optimism also helps dial down our
fear. 'Our mind, through design, will constantly look for the bad,'
Emma Murray told me. 'It will find the dirty floors, our overflowing laundry, our body shape, our underachieving kids, our
unsatisfying marriage, our poor performance at work, our lack of
friends, the things we should be doing but are not doing.'

The good news: we can train our brains to be optimistic. This
is where I reckon gratitude comes in—an attitude of gratitude can
truly improve your wellbeing. I am a big believer that to reframe
your outlook on things, you need to focus on haves, letting go
of have-nots. It's also a handy motivational tool, too. 'When you
focus on the goodness in your life, you create more of it,' as Oprah
says. Heard the saying 'neurons that fire together wire together?'
It's a neuroscience expression. It simply means you can change
the physiology of your brain through new thought patterns. Try
to notice the little things and truly appreciate them: the pay rise
albeit small, the hour at yoga, the short supermarket queue, the
positive twist in a conversation, or—look up—the sunshine.

Actually, there's a stack of research, Seligman's included, that's found that 'gratitude helps people feel more positive emotions, relish good experiences, improve their health, deal with adversity, and build strong relationships.' That quote comes from Harvard Medical School's beautifully titled mental health letter, *In Praise of Gratitude: Expressing thanks may be one of the simplest ways to feel better.* I'd also like to add in there (based on my own anecdotal evidence) that gratitude makes you feel more alive, sleep better and live with more compassion and kindness.

➤ *The Nectar List. Heard of it? It's a bit like a bucket list, but in reverse. Instead of listing things you want to do before you die, you write things you've already done—the achievements that have been the 'nectar' of your life thus far. I do it maybe once a year, looking back on that year and, my word, it's always a much-needed lesson in gratitude. Try it for yourself sometime.*

After seeing studies that recommended writing down three things you're grateful for every day, I tried it. For a month actually and, to be honest, it just became just another pesky thing to do. Instead, I gravitate to the advice I picked up a few years back in a book called *The Gratitude Diaries: How a year looking on the bright side transformed my life*, in which Janice Kaplan, journalist and former magazine editor, writes: 'Gratitude is long lasting and impervious to change or adversity. It requires an active emotional involvement—you can't be passively grateful, you actually have to stop and feel it, experience the emotion. So it creates an inner richness that's sustaining in difficult times as well as good ones.'

To me, gratitude—the art of appreciating what you have—is essential for a more balanced mental wellbeing.

WISDOM
KELLY CARTWRIGHT

Quick bio: Two little kids, two medals, two Paralympics, has climbed Mount Kilimanjaro once. Impressive. She lost her leg to a rare form of cancer when she was fifteen and is a passionate advocate for those living with a disability.

Interview need-to-know: She had me in tears the first time she spoke at a Women In Sport awards night. She's strong, fierce and kind. She hails from Geelong, so we spoke to each other over email.

Q: You're one of the most courageous and inspiring people I've met, what does the word courage mean to you?

A: Courage isn't always something you're born with. It's finding something inside yourself you didn't know existed until being courageous is your only choice. I believe it's when you step outside your comfort zone in order to grow and show yourself what you're capable of.

Q: Tell me about one of your most memorable 'stepping out of your comfort zone' moments.

A: I was asked to go on *Dancing With The Stars* in 2015 and my first reaction was, 'No way . . . I can't dance with one leg.' It's not very often I say I can't do something. But then I said to myself, *I want to show the world what people with disabilities are capable of and that we are all human.* I really had to dig deep to find the confidence and push my body really hard. I think I shocked myself the most—I proved to myself what I was truly capable of.

Q: How do you use this in your mum life as opposed to your sporting life?

A: Being a mum is tough! You doubt yourself some days and others you feel like you're so tired you'll fall asleep walking—you find courage and strength you didn't know you had when you become a mum. Believe in yourself first and foremost, believe that you can get through things, that's key.

Q: How do you cope today when you're feeling overwhelmed?

A: Some days I feel like I don't cope. And that's okay, but tomorrow is a new day, and through sport I learnt to take each day as it comes, focus on the little things and don't look too far into the future. Feeling overwhelmed comes with worrying about everything all at once. We are human and it's okay to take a step back and take a breath. Some days, I write down all the things I can control and all the things I can't—that puts into perspective what really matters.

Q: How we deal with our inner world drives everything in our outer world—how can we find the courage to face our fears?

A: Every situation is so different, but one thing that applies to all: surround yourself with the right people. Reach out to people who have gone through or are going through similar situations. You never have to go through anything alone, you can really learn from others' experience. I know I say this a lot: take each day as it comes, focus on the small positives that help drive you forward.

Q: What's your best piece of life advice for us?

A: Self-acceptance. We can get caught up in what we look like, what we wear, where we come from and how we should feel. Different is beautiful, it's powerful and it's okay being you . . . The confidence to own my leg, to wear it proudly, didn't come overnight—it took years to feel comfortable being different. As I realised I was making a difference to others' lives, I didn't want to cover my leg anymore. I wear it when I want and never go to the effort of covering it up. We get one life and I don't want to look back on mine and regret anything. Shoe shopping still sucks, but I can now wear heels.

Q: I also love the advice I read on your Instagram.

A: Oh yes, I don't believe things happen for a reason (I hate hearing that! Try telling someone who's lost someone this.) I believe shit just happens and it's how you deal with it that determines what is to come.

Q: You have great leadership in showing people that you can be enough just as you are . . .

A: Life needs to be more accessible—whether it's in the workforce, shopping centre or the everyday. I've felt out of place a lot in certain places. We all deserve the same lives, able-bodied or not.

Q: Your authenticity is on display beautifully in your Instagram posts . . .

A: There's not one mould, despite what you may see on social media. I want people to know that something can happen and be so terrible, but you can still come out the other side.

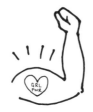

'I very much believe,
"Do what you're doing now
and do that well"—so just
fucking write a good email
now, and do a good column
now, and make that bit of
work right now good. Be
good in that meeting, show
up, do the work. And *then*
think about tomorrow.'

Zoë Foster Blake, author and cosmetics entrepreneur

CHAPTER TWELVE

OWN YOUR CONFIDENCE

It was a scorching early afternoon when I met Beyoncé in a Sydney bar with the Harbour Bridge commanding the view. The self-proclaimed feminist icon was fronting Destiny's Child back then; I was an eager upstart from a teen magazine (*Girlfriend*), busting with nerves. I'm sure she'd come across many young women like me.

Beyoncé was effortlessly cool yet poised—confident, too. I still recall the cheap vinyl black couch that suctioned my thighs every time I moved. (It was even more cringe-worthy to actually be able to hear it later when I transcribed the interview.) That night I stood right upfront at a VIP gig of 50 or so people listening to Destiny's Child's hits. I actually pulled out a picture of me with the band from that show recently—I'm snuggled between Beyoncé and Kelly Rowland—all of us, except Beyoncé, in leather jackets (mine fake) with long scarves. That look was so cool back then.

I posted that snap on my family's WhatsApp group (my brother-in-law, Phil, Lizie's husband, is a massive fan). I'll spare you the cheeky comments that came back. Looking back at my younger self, I seem so perfectly at home with my arms around three superstars—no one would've picked up that I was nervous as hell. Faking it, just like Beyoncé, as it turns out . . .

Beyoncé, to me, has always been the queen of confidence— proudly flying the feminist flag. (In fact, she confidently performed in front of a screen emblazoned with the word feminist—it was massive—during her Mrs Carter tour in 2016.) But even she admits she hasn't always been so sure of herself. I have since read that she was naturally shy and often felt intimidated at the beginning of her career, like when we first met (she fooled me!), hence the creation of her alter-ego Sasha Fierce, which she ceremoniously dumped in 2010. The confidence bit has taken her a lot of inner work to achieve.

I interviewed Beyoncé again a decade later, over the phone this time. I was more confident in my questioning and she didn't remember who I was, but then why would she—she was now a bona fide megastar. She still was friendly and chatty but talked with more force, more swagger in her voice.

In the words of Beyoncé: 'Your self-worth is determined by you.'

Mind you, Beyoncé might be the queen of owning it, but I have to share her vulnerability with you. In an *Elle* interview in 2019, one of their readers asked: 'What stresses you out? You always look like you're in control.' She replied:

I think the most stressful thing for me is balancing work and life. Making sure I am present for my kids—dropping Blue off at school, taking Rumi and Sir to their activities, making time for date nights with my husband, and being home in time to have dinner with my family—all while running a company can be challenging. Juggling all of those roles can be stressful, but I think that's life for any working mum.

Wow. It makes you realise that even for the Queen of Confidence, balance is bloody hard to achieve.

Confidence is a power tool

Be fierce. Be brave. Be bold. Own it. These mantras whirl around our world encouraging us to have confidence, be confident, own confidence . . . but, when you're weeping into your wine glass on a Friday night after everyone's tucked up in bed (or maybe that's just me when I am extra-exhausted) because you stuffed up at work, or you're freaking out about asking for a pay rise or finally calling out a lazy partner, watching TV while you're doing the mountain load of housework, these words can feel empty, like B.S.

I feel we often underplay the significant role confidence plays in how we attack life. Most of us struggle with confidence *daily,* whether it's work, body image, friendships or motherhood. Or just what to bloody wear. We also wrestle with that voice in our heads—*You sound stupid, You don't know what you're doing, You've got too much to do*—we get stressed and overwhelmed by it all and we're super hard on ourselves. The studies and stats back this up.

Having worked with hundreds of women, and dealing with my own stuff, I know this for a fact. Here's the thing: only 26 per cent of Australian women feel confident every day. This comes from a survey we did when we launched *whimn* in 2017. More than half of us—around 55 per cent—*frequently* experience self-doubt. Heck, our lives are a constant battle of internal conflicts and contradictions, so of course we question everything we do or don't do, everything we say or do not say, everything we want to do or do not want to do . . . I could go on. The *Dove Global Beauty and Confidence Report* from 2016 found that only 20 per cent of Australian women have high self-esteem.

In your toolkit of tricks to face down your overwhelm, confidence is a power tool. It's a glorious feeling of strength in yourself, in your truths, in your worth—it transforms wretched feelings of disempowerment (thanks again, mental load) into a sweet sense of empowerment. It's saying no; it's being disliked and being okay with that. It's pissing people off. It's failing, and then picking yourself up again; it's showing up. It's believing you can achieve, and knowing when to let go. Confidence gives you the power to withstand the dreadful times, the pride to trudge on, to push for change. It frees your mind from doubt, even just a little. You don't have to do it all, be it all—it's upwards and onwards with what's in front of you at the present moment. It gets you off the couch and into the world. Confidence can be a state of mind you arrive at throughout your day. Your confidence evolves. It's doing life your way, not how other people want, and being comfortable with your own insecurities. Confidence matters as much as competence— talent will get you so far, confidence propels you further.

'Confidence is the stuff that turns thoughts into action,' say Katty Kay and Claire Shipman in *The New York Times* bestseller *The Confidence Code*.

Here are a few things to ponder when putting confidence in your spotlight. First, it's about your self-worth—the value you place on yourself and your achievements (rather than comparing). It's self-assurance—a confidence in your own abilities free from doubt. And it's about moulding that self-esteem, your opinion of yourself, not so that you're better than others, but from a more secure place where comparison is irrelevant. I pulled this break- down from a cute book called *I Want To Be Confident* by Harriet Griffey as I thought it summed it up nicely.

Where do you find your confidence levels hover in these areas: self-worth, self-assurance and self-esteem? Nail what confid- ence means to you—'you do you'—and you will be better at riding the bumps, dealing with harsh stuff and not giving a shit about what other people think.

> ✑ 'It's about having confidence in who you are and what you stand for in any given moment—from the simple stuff, like when you have conflict with your partner, to the bigger decisions that will affect your team of twenty at work.'—*Lizie*

Bring your A game

Emma Murray uses a snappy technique I've since adopted on the home front, in my work and at the gym sometimes—so far, so good. She's all about bringing your A game instead of your B game. This is your A game: you're *aware* of your thoughts and feelings in the moment. You focus on your strengths and what you can bring to that moment: *I'm asking myself questions, I'm engaging in positive self-talk, I'm standing like this, holding myself like that.* In contrast, your B game is full of *what if, if only, it's not fair, I don't have enough time*-type thoughts. When you are focused on all the stuff out of your control, it leads to overwhelm.

We can't beat ourselves up for sitting in a B game state. Emma reassures me that it's a normal, natural human thing to do, and the more we accept we're biologically wired to sit in this headspace, the easier it is to shift out of it. Actually, we're wired to focus on the problems and the uncontrollables: it's the fight or flight response that's triggered so we can more quickly respond to danger. The longer we sit in this state (with today's open-ended stress, we literally never 'come down', our adrenalin forever firing), the more our brain adapts to it as the norm.

Dr Libby agrees, coming at it from a physiological point of view. 'It's catching these thoughts and beliefs that will ultimately alter our biochemistry, transform our health and our experience of stress, as well as how we live,' she tells me.

A game. Self-talk. It's all about confidence.

Recently my sister Ange posted a photo on Instagram that she took while she was rappelling off Mont Blanc in France for work (and I sit at a desk all day). She reminded me that our parents were big on the concept of growth mindset. They instilled the idea in each of their four kids that you don't have to *be* the best, you just need to *do* your best. If you put in the time and effort—and persevere—it leads to better, more fulfilling outcomes. When you're challenged, you grow. When you fail, you see it as a springboard to do better next time around.

➤ *Beware of the insidious power a simple selfie can have on your self-confidence. Psychologists at York University in Canada proved that selfies can destroy confidence, especially around body image. Those who took, edited and posted selfies on social media reported feeling less confident, more anxious and less physically attractive after the fact. It's easy to get lost in the ether of likes when you're asking for a stranger to (face) value you.*

In order to get a better grasp on this confidence thing, I enrolled myself in The School of Life's two-hour 'How To Be Confident' workshop. If you haven't heard about this place, it was set up in London by British philosopher and bestselling author Alain de Botton—their courses dig deep into emotional intelligence and what makes us tick.

There was a real mix of people at our Monday night workshop: ages 30 to 65, all nationalities, and plenty of women disorientated by their stress. As the strangers opened up about their confidence tussles, I felt I was sitting in one big therapy session. It was sympathetically reassuring. My nugget of wisdom to share with you from it: your inner voice is the key to confidence. I'm a big believer in empowering self-talk—it has a stunning power to shift how you think, feel and behave. You need to allow your inner voice to be compassionate, like a best buddy, a cheerleader, your go-to guide, like someone you would give a big squeezy bear hug to, someone you like, actually, no—someone you love. You need to consciously tune into it (hello awareness!), acknowledge it and call it the hell out when it gets nasty, unkind or destructive. And if you screw up or mess up, tell yourself it isn't so bad and encourage yourself to give it another go. The sun will rise and you can try again tomorrow.

As I've been writing this part of the book, I've been clocking the words I tell myself throughout my days (running from work to school pick-up to supermarket to home; while exercising, at home and so on). The ones I like best: *I can do this, you got this, keep going, you'll get there, you'll feel better afterwards, you're at the bottom of the U!* All these weave in and out of my thoughts and they have an uncanny knack of lessening the stress, easing the anxiety and buffering my outlook with optimism.

Good self-talk can be simple, like switching your pronouns. A bunch of US psychology professors found a pronoun can help you psych yourself up when faced with more intense life stuff. 'We found that cueing people to reflect on intense emotional experiences using their names and non-first-person pronouns such as "you" or "he" or "she" consistently helped them control their thoughts, feelings, and behaviors,' wrote two of the professors in the *Harvard Business Review*. They used a powerful example to explain it. When the Nobel Prize–winner Malala Yousafzai found out she was on the Taliban's hit list, she told US talk show host Jon Stewart she was fearful (as you bloody well would be), but then she visualised how she'd respond if she was attacked: 'I said, "If he comes, what would you do, Malala?" . . . Then I would reply [to] myself, "Malala, just take a shoe and hit him."'

One psychologist I interviewed years ago had another trick: those negative thoughts in the background? Think of them as your kids making a ruckus in the back seat when you're focusing on driving. Ignore, ignore, ignore.

There's a tonne of research about the power of positive self-talk, but I don't need to bore you with those semantics as it's just a case of trying it on for size. I'm no pro at this, I'm just like you—remembering and reminding, being gentle on myself, too. When I go on TV each week to dissect the news of the day, I am talking to myself way before I walk on set—I'm telling myself, *You know what to say, if not wing it, otherwise nail it.* Look, sometimes I do and other times I fluff it. When I can't be arsed exercising, I tell myself, *But think of how you'll feel afterwards.* When I have a thorny work email that needs a reply, I say to myself, *Let's write this slowly, be wise with your words.* When I've got a particularly wild-looking week looming, I remind myself with self-talk that I will get through.

My husband's also an advocate of this whole self-talk thing and he calls it the self-talk cycle. Before a game of footy, Tom would jot down this little formula in his special book: self-talk, self-image, performance. Talk yourself up and you'll project a positive self-image and, in turn, your performance will reflect someone in control. And vice versa. Then he'd read it just before he ran from the change rooms and onto the field.

Motherhood's a clincher for wreaking havoc on self-talk, isn't it? We just can't help but compare, question and doubt. Blimey, even Kate Middleton confessed she struggled with confidence when she first became a mum. Actually, when my first baby came along, it was one of the most challenging times for my confidence levels. Breastfeeding in public petrified me, going to the supermarket was a nightmare (who says wiping shit off yourself thanks to your son having a mighty big explosion in Woolies isn't confidence building? I've tried it) and turning up to that first mothers' group? Oh boy. And then there's returning to work, too.

Fronting up to then PM Julia Gillard asking for money for our 'I Support Women In Sport' awards . . . well, that took an extra big dose of positive self-talk. I often wonder if I had more confidence when I was younger. Sometimes, I think we all do. Confidence ebbs and flows throughout life, always at the mercy of the curve balls we're thrown.

Just to make you feel a tad better about all this, there are evolutionary wirings that stroke our self-doubt (I'm beginning to feel the brain is often not on our side). I'll leave this to neuropsychologist Judy Ho, who wrote about this in *Psychology Today*, to explain:

> The source of self-sabotage is part of a common ancestral and evolutionary adaptation. We are essentially programmed to strive for goals because achieving them makes us feel good. That dopamine rush is an incentive to repeat those behaviors. The trick, especially when it comes to self-sabotage, is that our biochemistry doesn't necessarily discriminate between the kind of feel-good sensations we experience when we are going toward our

goals and the 'good' feelings we get when we avoid something that seems threatening.

Damn that brain again.

Be fierce in your self-talk. Practice bringing your A game. It works.

> ✒ 'I never thought I was good enough to be a photographer up
> with the boys, but I didn't let it become a barrier. I just focused
> on learning what I didn't know and then practising it over
> and over. I showed my worth by not only being the hardest
> worker out there, but also by striving to be the best I can at
> my craft.'—*Ange*

Be brave against doubt

Not sure if you remember, but back in Chapter Five, I mentioned my neighbour Jen. She tried for kids for years, had a daughter in her forties through IVF, and sold her successful clothing business in order to raise her. Her husband runs a construction company, so she carries the main chunk of the mental load. 'When you're in your early twenties everything is at your fingertips—you can earn a decent wage—but now it's different. I'm 49 and I'm unemployable. Or I have to take a lesser role for less money, and have to leave to pick up my daughter,' Jen tells me. Might I add, she was the well-known voice of a national radio station years ago, ran that successful clothing business and has many transferable skills. I remind her of that famous Tina Fey quote: 'Confidence is 10 per cent hard work and 90 per cent delusion—just thinking foolishly that you will be able to do what you want to do.' Fake it until you make it, indeed. But Jen's lack of confidence reminds me it's a common feeling, especially when you return to work after mat leave, when the impostor syndrome kicks in, the guilt and—pfft—there go your boundaries.

At The School of Life course, they referred to self-sabotage as 'an attempt to bring our external reality back in line with what we feel we inwardly deserve'. Scarily, the very next week after my chat with Jen, a US study popped up in my inbox which proved that if a woman suffers impostor syndrome at work (hello, yes, 99 per cent of us, according to my quick straw poll of friends), they in turn suffer from emotional exhaustion, which leads to more conflict between work and family life *and* less satisfaction at work. Can we really win?

'Confidence is a real bugbear of mine,' Emma Murray says when I quiz her on whether she suffers impostor syndrome working in a hugely successful male-dominated footy club—she does! 'When you ask most women they would say, but she's confident—I'm not. Gee, I wish I was like that. Confidence is not a personality trait, confidence is a skill, a tool—it's something we learn. We need to redefine confidence as a willingness to try. Take a step to actually have a willingness to try.' I like that concept—a willingness to try.

Sheryl Sandberg has also tackled confidence:

Confidence and leadership are muscles. You learn to use them or you learn not to. If you are afraid to speak up at a meeting, every time you force yourself to do it, you get better at it. If you're afraid to take your seat at the table, every time you take your seat at the table and you realise no one tells you to go get back to the back row, you learn to do it.'

It's no wonder so many of us suffer loss of confidence when returning to work after mat leave—apart from anything else, we're out of practice at the kind of confidence you build every day at work.

So, there's this thing, too, called the confidence/competence loop. Which comes first, confidence or competence? The more competent you are doing a particular thing, the more confident you will be, but the reverse is also true. Because our subconscious mind reverts to fear (which means no action) when we get nervous, doubt creeps in and we procrastinate. When you push past the fear, you take action, your mind goes, *Oh, that was okay, I'll try again based on the learning I got from that first time* and it allows us to take another step and another step. Remember this the next time you're doing something that scares the shit out of you.

- 'When I embarked on a new gig in digital media a couple of years ago, everything changed. I felt like I had to read the whole internet before bed just to keep on top of it all. I started drinking a lot of coffee to get powered up and a good slug of red wine at night to get back down. This went on for twelve months before I got some professional help. Those were some dark times, but I'm really proud of myself for bouncing back. Sometimes all it takes is having the confidence to put your hand up and ask for help.'—*Ash*

- 'In those soul-crushing moments of defeat I take one moment at a time. When it's −40 degrees at work shooting an Olympic skier, the wind howling and my eyelashes are frozen shut, I focus only on the most pressing challenge at hand. Rather than getting overwhelmed or distracted by the many other challenges in my periphery.'—*Ange*

Be bold in your living #ownit

It's ironic, really, that when I'm deep into writing this chapter, I have a mini-crisis of confidence of sorts. Weird, but human I suppose. I suddenly become really self-critical of the words on this page—a nonsensical self-sabotage. It's suffocating—an implosion of stress—based mostly on doubt and fear. So, I have a cry to myself on the couch (no one else is home), and then do exactly what the research says we all do: I procrastinate.

I walk up the road—justifying this on the grounds that 'motion changes emotion' (thanks Emma)—to grab some groceries and stop into my local bookshop on the way back. As I am fangirling Elizabeth Gilbert at this point in my life, I reach for her non-fiction book *Big Magic: Creative living beyond fear.* It's the only one of hers I haven't read. I flick open the book and, I kid you not, it lands on this subheading: 'Done Is Better Than Good'. It's a sign. And just like that, I've stopped the silly negative self-talk and my confidence is back.

(There's a stellar quote Elizabeth uses from US Army General George Patton: 'A good plan violently executed now is better than a perfect plan executed next week.' Her take: 'A good-enough novel violently written now is better than a perfect novel meticulously written never.' Works for anything in life—done is better than perfect, indeed.)

Risk-taking is a big part of strengthening confidence, isn't it? Of course, we're risk averse, not wanting to fail, look silly, place ourselves in danger, jeopardise our life savings . . . I could go on. The risks don't have to be huge—or crazy—to build our confidence. I came across a neat little term called 'stretching', it's almost an updated word version of 'take the risk', and a little less scary in some ways. It comes from a book called *The Power of Moments* by two US university professors, brothers Chip and Dan Heath. In it, they write: 'To stretch is to place ourselves in situations that expose us to the risk of failure.' They use a lovely example of a woman, Lea, 42, who took a risk opening a bakery but became so overwhelmed with this on top of the rest of her life, she had to close it. You could say she technically failed, but as they put it: 'In the process she learned more about her capabilities and her values . . . the promise of stretching is not success, it's learning.'

> ⬊ *There's merit to that pesky meme—'Should have. Could have. Would have. Did'—even if it doesn't work out. Take the risk! Take on a project at work that scares the bejesus out of you just to prove to yourself you can. Do something on your own, so you can raise a glass to yourself afterwards.*

I came across a hashtag not so long ago: #appropriatelyconfident. It was started by obstetrician and long-term questioner of the validity of Goop's health advice, Dr Jennifer Gunter (she also wrote that book, *The Vagina Bible*), and was a call to women to share the shit they're good at. Women jumped on, slowly, and when I read them I (almost) fist-pumped the air. I'll share my fave: 'I'm fat. I'm beautiful. I'm worthy of love. I matter. My size doesn't validate any of this.' That one gave me goosebumps. Made me a little teary, too (tears galore in this chapter). Oh, and one more: 'I am an amazing baker. I make delicious things. Also, I made uterus cookies and brought them to the hospital for the docs and nurses the day of my hysterectomy.' Funny.

The editor of *whimn*, Melissa Shedden, wrote a piece about the hashtag and opened up about when she's downplayed her successes or censored herself. I especially love this bit she wrote:

As women, we're encouraged to shrink not just our bodies on public transport, but our achievements, so we take up less room, allowing men the space to succeed. But #appropriatelyconfident is one of those new Twitter campaigns that wants to give the two-finger salute to this patriarchal hangover . . . It's only appropriate we be confident—for ourselves, and each other.

Why, as women, do we do this? If you feel there's something you have a strength in, hold tight to it and share it. You don't have to shout it in an arrogant or boastful way—you can be polite, modest and gentle. You can be humble enough to know your limitations. Play to your strengths, strengthen your strengths and focus on what you can bring to the situation. However, it's also about not overdoing things or overcommitting just to prove your worth. Own up to what you do well (at work), stand up for yourself (at home), draw the line (with yourself) and don't apologise for who you are (with others). Now I am sure Beyoncé would recommend that.

WISDOM
TURIA PITT

Quick bio: Inspiration to every Australian woman. Can I just leave it at that? Why not. (Sidenote: mum, author of *Everything To Live For*, *Unmasked* and *Good Selfie*, humanitarian, athlete and motivational speaker).

Interview need-to-know: She lives near my parents, but once again life got in the way of my wish of sharing a long beach walk and dissecting life. All I can say is, thank the heavens for email.

Q: How do you deal with feeling overwhelmed in life?

A: Feeling overwhelmed is just part of the deal, right? *breathes into a paper bag* My favourite tip is to stop looking at the big picture. I know that sounds counterintuitive, but when you're constantly looking at the enormity of the task ahead, it's easy to feel demoralised, because the gap between where you are and where you want or need to be is so big. It can feel impossible to manage. Keep focused on the task today. Don't worry about tomorrow, or what you have to do 'next'. Just focus on the small step you can take today.

Q: I love your idea of the 'overwhelm list'—talk me through that.

A: I first heard about this via Marie Forleo (life coach, motivational speaker, author and web television host of *MarieTV*). Grab a piece of paper and write down absolutely everything that's renting space in your head; that's all you have to do—write it down. Set a timer for ten minutes, just so it doesn't feel overwhelming in itself. This part in itself is super therapeutic. There's something about physically writing it down that is calming, as opposed to it being a nonstop, repetitive loop of panic in your head. Then, you examine your list. Anything that's outside of your control, like the weather for the party you've organised or wanting your boss to like you, cross off your list. Next, cross off all the 'shoulds'. You know, the things you keep telling yourself you should do but don't actually want to do—like catching up with that old colleague or joining the P&C at your kid's school. The only items left on your list now should be things you have to do, want to do or actually can do—the stuff that you can control. Now you can prioritise these, schedule them and get them done. Outsource some tasks. Like the cake you wanted to make for your sister's birthday but don't have time for? Guess who is calling the bakery tomorrow? You are.

Q: In your book *Good Selfie*, you say confidence is the thing you're asked about most. What's your secret?

A: Not relying solely on one aspect of yourself for your confidence—for a lot of people there's this perception that the 'better' we look, the more confidence we'll have. Now, there's nothing wrong with presenting the best version of yourself to the world. I love rocking fresh threads, getting my make-up done, exploring new medical advancements to smooth my skin etc. When I rock up for a speech or interview or meeting having taken pride in my appearance, I feel more capable and confident. BUT don't fall into the massive trap of thinking your appearance is the only facet that determines your confidence. Because confidence comes from LOTS of different things. For me that includes my physical fitness, surrounding myself with people who make me feel good, how well my business is growing and performing (and how much I'm learning) and my involvement in fundraising and helping my community.

Q: How do you tame your inner critic?

A: Everyone has an inner critic. And by everyone, I mean every single human on this planet. LeBron James, Oprah, Beyoncé—everyone's got one. And what our inner critic does is make us feel like we're not enough. We're not smart enough to take on that project, we're not dedicated enough to finish that digital course we just bought, we're not attractive enough to ask that hottie for their number, we're not creative or talented or smart or productive or whatever . . . the bottom line is the same: we're not 'enough' to live the life we want for ourselves.

Q: So, how do your curb the negative self-talk?

A: Be your own bestie. I mean, would you ever speak to a friend the way you speak to yourself? If your partner had a rough day at the office, would you say, 'Yeah, you are a failure'? Would you sit down with your daughter after she lost a running race and say, 'Why did you even bother, you're crap at running anyway'? If your girlfriend rang you and was upset about a mistake she made at work, would you say, 'Well, you always do fuck things up'. Next time you catch that negative mental loop, think about how you would talk to someone you love. Instead of saying, 'Yeah, you are lazy and you've dropped the ball', say, 'It's okay mate, everyone makes mistakes. You're human! And this feeling won't last.' Remember: you can either be your own worst enemy or your greatest ally.

Q: Why do you think confidence for women is so important to making sense of our crazy-busy lives?

A: We all want to feel confident, and loved, and like we're making progress in our lives. At the end of the day, we all want to look back on the things we've done and think, *Shit yeah, I did THAT.*

Q: Your confidence has enabled you to achieve great things— what's been the one area it's helped you most and how?

A: It absolutely helps in all areas of life, but particularly in business it's critical. Say you have two people who are identical in terms of their abilities. One of those people is pessimistic, has a negative mindset and doesn't have faith in themselves. The other person backs themselves, believes in themselves and has a positive mindset. It's pretty obvious which person will experience more success!

And more than that, the person with the negative mindset will perceive failures (which are inevitable, both professionally and personally!) to be a confirmation of their lack of ability. The person with the positive mindset, however, will perceive the failure to be a learning opportunity for what they can do differently next time.

Q:　What does wellness mean to you?

A:　Wellness means looking after yourself—mentally and physically. Getting enough sleep, moving your body, drinking enough water and eating real food, hanging out with people who make you feel good about yourself and keeping your self-talk positive and strong. And it's also about making time for the things that make you happy, and setting challenges for yourself. Most of all, it's a process—not a destination. Because you're not gonna get it all right, all the time. And that's okay.

Q:　What do you do that brings you a sense of wellbeing in your life?

A:　I'm pretty big on my morning routine and I never used to be a morning person! But I find that if I spend five or ten minutes getting my mind right before I start my day, everything is easier. I actually even made a little Morning Mindset Routine mini-course for people who want to get their mornings powering too. A big part of that routine is practising gratitude—it's a game changer. I keep it really simple—I wake up, open the blinds, wake up Hakavai (let's be real, he's usually the one waking me up). I set him up with some toys while I make a coffee and then sit while I watch him play.

Q: Ahhh coffee, the first thing I am always grateful for.

A: I think of three things I'm really, truly grateful for. As soon as I start focusing on what I'm grateful for, I can feel my body respond. I'm more conscious of my heart beating, of the way my breath fills and expands my lungs. Positive images start flooding my brain and my perspective shifts. It's the best way to start your day. And it's the easiest and quickest way to short-circuit negative feelings throughout the day, too. It's an antidote to envy, bitterness, anger, hostility, boredom, fear, shame, humiliation. I mean, think about it, it's impossible to be grateful and angry at the same time, or grateful and bitter at the same time. When you're truly grateful that's the only emotion you'll experience. Pretty cool, huh?

'Faith, family and friends provide the scaffolding on which I build my life.'

Sheena Percival (aka my mum)

CHAPTER THIRTEEN

THE POWER OF CONNECTION

It's a cruel irony that literally the day I begin this chapter, disaster strikes my family and I'm reminded of the unpredictability of life.

It's around 9.30 on New Year's Eve morning 2019 when Mum calls me from my parents' home in the quaintly colourful coastal town of Lake Conjola on the New South Wales South Coast. It's one of those breezy 'I'm just calling to check in' kind of chats. I'm learning to treasure those more as she's getting older. As I hang up, I wish her a Happy New Year.

At 11 a.m. I get a text from my sister Ange, who is with them: 'Bushfires raging, we're loading the car with the photo albums.' Tom switches on the TV—reports say the fire is fierce and hurtling towards Lake Conjola. Why didn't Mum mention this? Around midday, as I am struggling to hold a too-full basket in the bustling supermarket with one son in tow, Dad calls, flustered. He is running, puffing. 'There's fire all around us, we're alright . . .' The phone line crackles, then goes dead.

This is almost my undoing.

The next six hours are an agonising wait as I trawl every possible source for information. All power and phone lines are burnt out. Mid-afternoon, we finally get a flurry of WhatsApp messages from Ange: safe, actually in the water off the beach and choking in smoke. She sends a video, too. The wind is howling, the fire hurtling towards them, spot fires sparking only metres away, as helicopters scoop up hundreds of litres of water from the lake and dump them on the fire.

I will never forget this bit of my sister's message: 'I could see the flames from the living room window . . . where do I find Dad? . . . picking TOMATOES. Clearly that's when I started yelling. I stayed very calm, then I yelled, then I cried. I have never experienced anything like that level of emergency. One minute we were packing the Esky, the next we were running for our lives.' (Remember, this is the sister who rappels down the face of ice cliffs for work, for goodness sake.)

I jump on a Facebook group, a godsend for those on the outside desperate to connect with those on the inside, trying to find out if they are free from injury and if their house is still standing. I chat on the phone with complete strangers, Mum and Dad's neighbours, through tears and nervous laughter. The human spirit is a magnificent thing.

Our parents' house was spared, unlike nearly 100 others in the tiny town. With only one road in and out, they were trapped for three days with no power, no supplies and no real idea of the destruction and risk still around them—like a war zone, Mum told me later.

I hugged Mum, Dad and Ange so tightly when we reconnected—reassuring each other that the most important thing in life was us. We're built to support, connect and rally in tough times, aren't we?

The curve ball of the bushfires was loaded with another timely message: friends and family show up when you fall in a heap, they stand beside you, they listen. I received so many simple, yet compassionate texts.

And, as we theorised later, picking his tomatoes was simply Dad's way of dealing with the hysteria—everyone has different coping mechanisms. That's good to remember too.

The key to healthy wellbeing

So, here's the ultimate secret to living a good life, an enriched life, a well life, a more balanced one: true wellness is about deep, healthy, empowering connections with your partner, kids, family, friends, colleagues and community. Connections with people. We are more connected with people than ever before—look at how invaluable a phone and internet connection was in the drama of the fires—but so often our screen connection isn't real. The emotion can be misread, the power of face-to-face human interaction lost. Digital distraction wreaks havoc on our tired brains. We hide behind our screens and avoid true connection. We kid ourselves that we're connected, when really, we're not.

As far back as 530 BC, Pythagoras (the ancient triangle theory guy) nailed it: 'Friends are as companions on a journey, who ought to aid each other to persevere in the road to a happier life.'

So, let's stop our tribes shrinking, prevent friendships from falling away and neighbours being nobodies—make the effort. Go for dinner, invite them over. Do something good and, in turn, you'll feel good and so the cycle begins.

Often when we're breathless in our days, suffocated by mental loads, drowning in responsibilities and hung up on expectations, our relationships are the first thing to slip down the list of priorities. When, in fact, they should be right up the top. *Oh, but I'm so exhausted, there is no flippin' way I can meet her for dinner tonight.* And then you sprawl on the couch watching *Married At*

First Sight. Come on, we're all guilty of this one. Or this: 'I am too busy to call' and then you sit on social media for fifteen minutes in a wet towel before pulling on your PJs.

I admit I feel like a bit of a fraud writing this, because too often I've blown off a drinks invitation, failed to call my best mate back for days, not phoned a friend lost in grief or let the guilt consume me for missing someone's birthday . . . all because life is too busy, too hectic, I have too much going on. I, too, am remorseful for 'skimming on all my important relationships', as a friend once lamented to me.

It's too easy to take our good relationships for granted too often—*Oh, she'll understand if I don't go.* In fact, relationships with friends, family and partners—the healthy ones, that is—can be much-needed therapy for your stress, an antidote to your overwhelm and exhilarating for the soul. Kemi told me: 'It's easy to forget how important the people close to you are, we often ignore them over the bright shiny object things, whatever they are.' How true.

It's simple evolution, really—we're designed to form close bonds, to exist in a pack. Back when we hung out in caves with bones in our hair, we survived in our tribe so we could hunt animals, protect each other, share water—and those fundamentals have not changed. In fact, researchers say we're hardwired to connect: that spending quality time with others is as important to us as water and sleep.

Social researcher Hugh Mackay says: 'Most of us define the meaning of our lives in terms of our relationships, and our relationships define us. Unless we nurture these connections through communication, they lose their significance for us—which is another way of saying we lose something of ourselves.'

Loneliness, for example, has been linked to a plethora of health problems, from high blood pressure to cancer to weaker immunity. One study concluded that loneliness can, quite literally, hurt your heart. It kills. Social belonging also brings an enriching sense of purpose and identity. One of the world's longest running studies out of Harvard Univesity—that has now clocked in at more than 80 years—has seen researchers tag-teaming and following a group of men, at first, and now their wives. (Just as well.) The big question they asked: what keeps people happy and healthy throughout their lives? The critical finding was that meaningful relationships are the number one predictor of health, happiness and longevity. Sure, genes and caring for your body count, but connection is like a shield, the protector through life's rougher times.

> ⊠ There's a TEDx Talk on this called 'What Makes a Good Life: Lessons from the longest study on happiness'. . . if you ever find a spare hour.

Sure, the research is there, but my own sobering experience has gently reaffirmed it. I was sitting at my desk one day when my grandfather called me to tell me that my grandmother's life was nearing the end. She was 92 and had lived, in her words, 'a good life'. My sister Eliza and I hotfooted it to the hospital. When I walked into the darkened room, Marnie, as we called her, was lying eerily still, cords like spaghetti around her bed. I held her hand, stroked her arm—her skin felt like tissue paper. I walked into the bathroom and looked at myself in the mirror, teary-eyed and my heart as heavy as concrete. I said to myself, *This is the last time you will talk to your grandmother alive.*

I perched on the side of her bed, held her hand and asked her this: 'What's one piece of wisdom you can share, the most important thing you've learnt in your life?' She answered in a hushed, puffed whisper.

'Take care of the people closest to you, as that is all that really matters in life. That you are all close to me now—that's a life worth living.'

The art of friendship

I tell you what also makes a life worth living—a close connection with someone who understands, who listens, who values and who responds without judgement, just with love. Or hugs. And wine, when you need it. A friend who just shows up, stands up whenever you need . . . as you do for them.

Glennon Doyle, author of bestseller *Love Warrior*, sums this up beautifully: 'This back-and-forth is repeated again and again as we go deeper into each other's hearts, minds, pasts, and dreams. Eventually, a friendship is built—a solid, sheltering structure that exists in the space between us—a space outside of ourselves that we can climb deep into. There is her, there is me, and then there is our friendship—this bridge we've built together.'

A sheltering structure, that's exactly what we need.

When my eldest son was in preschool, I made a new best friend, a rare occurrence as you get older, I think. First, our kids became buddies and then I officially met 'the mum', Dana, at the beginning of their first year at school. She had a warm smile, effervescent energy and a strong Canadian accent—which made it easy for us to start those initial conversations, as I'd lived there myself (and my sister still does). We are the same age and have the same juggles in life—career, family, marriage. We share the same feminist ideals and, the best bit, we both agree that balance is B.S.! Of course we had to be friends! She's a teacher, and now a friendship expert and founder of URSTRONG, a social and emotional wellbeing program for kids. Basically, she teaches children how to form and maintain healthy, vibrant friendships. Her inspiration for her business was when she noticed women were constantly pitted against each other in pop culture—*Real Housewives*, *The Bachelor*—and even more disturbingly, in children's shows like *Barbie* and *My Little Pony*. Thanks to her appetite for statistics and research, she's a pro at this for adults too.

'Good friendships can benefit our mental health in so many ways: friends reduce stress, make us laugh, help us feel known and understood, motivate us to take care of ourselves and reach higher, and fulfil the basic need of belonging,' she tells me while tucking into her acai bowl one day after the kids have finished school. 'Positive relationships are the top protective factor against depression, anxiety and other mental health disorders.'

Sharing your true thoughts, your hurt, pain, your ups and downs is an incredibly healing and therapeutic thing to do, even if your friend doesn't have any answers. Which they most likely won't. But just think—they might suggest an alternative way to tackle something that's bothering you. Sure, it takes strength and courage to open up to your friends, but the pay-off is better than any wellness cure. It lifts your spirit. It feeds your soul.

I often feel nostalgic for my early twenties, when friends were the centre of my universe—oh, and my career. When *Sex and the City* and *Friends* reminded me that life was pure fun. And *Dawson's Creek* (where Joey Potter was everyone's wannabe best friend). And then you hit 30, or you have kids, or your friends do, and it gets trickier to fit it all in. There is no time! We have no mental space!

You know, this could also be our own doing. 'Women have this polished facade and don't always talk about what's really going on,' Dana texts me late one night. 'When we hit a certain age there are more things you *don't* talk about than things you do—a barrier snaps up and you're only sharing what's appropriate. When you're single and dating, you're way more open—"How are things going with your boyfriend?"—a super normal question. "How are things going with your husband?"—a super inappropriate question. For this reason, I wonder if women feel bottled up? It comes back to pressure around having to portray the perfect life, but the feeling of being "bottled up" is isolating and is not good.'

This is a reminder for me: real friendship needs to go beyond surface chats, which can be hard in a world full of #squadgoals and juggling boyfriends or girlfriends, partners and kids. It's hard to unmask how you're really feeling—to admit you're lonely, you're not coping, you can't see your way through or you need help. The mums' group I joined after the birth of my first son has always been an unequivocal support in this sense.

'The greatest barriers to connection are within us,' writes Hugh Mackay. In our world of 256 Facebook friends, we need quality over quantity—'feel-good friendships' as Dana calls them—and we need to keep 'focusing on what works'. We need at least one friendship deeply rooted in trust and respect. The 'poo friend' as I once heard it called in my office: that one friend you can talk to about absolutely anything . . . even the colour of your shit. I have three of these friends (two formed in my twenties and now Dana as well); you may have five and that's okay too. 'There's a lot of research that talks about the power of vulnerability in forming close connections,' Dana adds. 'But you can only be vulnerable with someone if trust and respect are at the core of your friendship—you can confide in them, feel comfortable and you can be yourself. Ultimately, you feel seen and heard and valued.'

Shasta Nelson, author of *Frientimacy*, reckons there are three factors that must work together to achieve a close connection: positivity, vulnerability and consistency. Friendships take effort . . . and I get it, it's hard to fit them in. There are tricks to it: think about things you already do and where friend time could seamlessly fit in. Lock them down for a wine on the weekend and just sit and listen, *really listen*, to them talking and actually hear what they are saying. Ask more questions, and often you will get, and give, a deeper answer. What a wonderful way to lighten the mental load . . . even if it's just for a night.

It's even harder to make time to work at friendships that have hit a bump in the road. Dana is great on this. She has developed the concept of 'Friendship Fires'—common conflicts that exist in all relationships. Of course, this is a cute term usually reserved for her presentations, where she takes schoolkids through a step-by-step guide on how to face conflict rather than avoid it. But I reckon this applies to adults, too. (Sidenote: Dana tells me she's often inundated with requests from mums after their daughters' seminars, asking for help with their own lives.)

Timeworn sentiments like 'Just ignore her!', 'She's just jealous!' and 'Suck it up!' have turned us into master conflict-avoiders, and this is when resentment and aggression take root. These 'fires' get bigger and bigger until someone explodes. Have you had one of those blow-ups? Me too. 'When we face conflict head-on in our friendships, we create deeper roots of trust and respect. Our friendship gets stronger and closer because we know each other better and we got through it together,' Dana tells me.

On one hand it's damn hard to make friends and maintain solid friendships as an adult; on the other it's hard to let go of unhealthy friends and relationships that are draining your well-being. Pink has a swell way of saying it. 'Edit your friendships. As you get older you definitely have less time,' she wrote on her Instagram. '1. Feel reciprocal. 2. Don't drain your life force. 3. Fill your tank with love and good energy.' Love that.

> ⟍ *I like to think of friendship as a verb—this means 'friends' actually call or text or drop over or make you soup. They don't post a pic with a hashtag and call it a day—remember, their actions (and yours) speak louder than words.*

After talking to all the experts in this book, I get a sense that all these wise women are strategic about who they let into their lives—they guard their time. Kemi nailed it for me: 'I'm committed to being with women who are honest—there is no comparison or competing. I have a very small inner circle and we are allowed to put on the table the real stuff that's going on. It's non-judgemental, we don't give advice unless we're asked for it. And it's just like, can you be with me right now while we're experiencing life together?' Being true to yourself matters, because if you're not, it's just another thing in your mental load, right? I think so. 'We curate who we get to be in certain spaces for fear of being discarded,' she added. 'You know our ultimate fear is being kicked out of the tribe. We spend a lot of energy making sure that we belong to the side, but are you clear on the tribe you want to belong to?'

> ⟍ 'Hanging out in my mums' group once a week helps me to face the world—and all the bullshit we, as women, wade through each day—with more courage and more clarity. Connecting

with like-minded, supportive women helps me recharge and reset for the week to come.'—*Lizie*

When friendship meets feminism

Feminism is about equal rights for women, friendship is about valuing and supporting each other—combine the two and let them feed off each other, and it's an almighty force. Women lifting each other up, giving each other voice. Since women's marches took over the globe as part of the #MeToo movement, the importance of rallying with and for other women is at an all-time high.

The next wave of feminism is here and, my lordy, it's a beautifully intoxicating thing. Back in 2014, in her brilliant collection of essays, *Bad Feminist*, Roxane Gay called out this point perfectly— don't be an enemy, be an ally: 'Abandon the cultural myth that all female friendships must be bitchy, toxic, or competitive. This myth is like heels and purses—pretty but designed to *slow* women down.'

I truly feel we, as women, are going through a real shift— we're abandoning this myth in force. We're being less competitive (*The Bachelor* days might be numbered), more willing to help, support, work together; to be more tolerant, accepting and kinder. Yes, kindness is cool. Perhaps many of us now finally realise the secret weapon that is actually #womensupportingwomen. In a recent US poll, 79 per cent of respondents reported that they believed women are supporting women now more than ever before. Do you?

So, here's the thing: while this is all ramping up in our workplaces, on the streets and in society as a whole and we're shifting little by little, we still need to make sure we're supporting each

other's wellbeing in our own communities. Right now. Today. We
need to move beyond our social media hashtags, we need to walk
the talk.

On about our fifth 'friend date', Dana and I went to see
Belgian psychotherapist Esther Perel. You know her? Now living
in NYC, Perel's fly-on-the-wall, frank therapy sessions in her
office have made her a worldwide podcast sensation. Add *Where
Should We Begin* to your to-listen-to list, it really is that good.

She said one thing during her talk that stuck with both of us.
She highlighted the importance of calling people, because hearing
someone's voice is like hearing music—it provides a deeper
connection. It worries Esther that we don't just pick up the phone
anymore. The speed of life and technology have broken down our
communities and we don't have the strength around us that we
did in the past, that village mentality. At the end of the day, who's
going to feed your cat? she asked us. Who's going to help you
when everyone else has forgotten?

'I have been thinking a lot about this,' said Dr Rebecca
Huntley when we talked about what true wellness really means.
'One of the issues around wellness is there is a limit to how much
you can do as an individual. Unless we have a community-wide
approach to physical and mental health, wellness isn't achievable.
I think about the times in my life when I've been really stretched,
it's always been a combination of me taking control of my own
health but having friends and support around to do that and living
in a community where that's possible.' We need a society that
creates breathing space for people to connect. The more you make
it about the individual, the harder relationships are to maintain.

This connection can be as small as a micro-moment, those
quick connections you make with not just friends, but workmates,
the bloke in your coffee queue, the young girl also walking

her dog. Often these conversations might feel superficial, a bit ho-hum, but if you put in a little effort and tune in, they can become so much more in terms of your wellbeing.

A leading US researcher on happiness and positive emotions, psychologist and author Barbara Frederickson, found that these micro-moments can give you an oxytocin hit—you know, the feel-good hormone. They take you outside yourself, albeit briefly.

When Tom and I travelled through Central America on our honeymoon, we stopped in Cuba first. In the dilapidated town of Cienfuegos, we stayed with a middle-aged man called Alberto and his equally vibrant wife (it's all homestays out of Havana). We literally checked in at 9 p.m. and left at 9 a.m. and as he couldn't speak much English our interactions involved a lot of hand movements. Alberto had a brightness in his face, a friendliness in his speech; energy to his life. To this day, I can still remember how good that brief connection made me feel. A micro-moment, that's all you need—to not only make someone's day, but leave an imprint for life.

Easy to tune in to this when you're on holidays, you'll say, without a care in the world. But if you pay a bit more attention and pause for a moment to appreciate the small things, you'll start to recognise the oxytocin hit when a little boy comes running after you in the park with your baby's favourite toy; when a young woman in the coffee queue tucks your dress tag in with a knowing smile. And you'll never forget the kind lady who leans over on the train and says quietly, 'Honey, you've got toothpaste in your hair.'

I used to wish they would bottle oxytocin and sell it on the black market, so good is this hormone's uncanny way of injecting a lift into your day. But it's free anyway, and it works both ways. Appreciate the small moments and then pass them on.

⤴ 'I have only a few business besties and a ten-minute chat
changes the whole course of the week—surrounding yourself
with like-minded friends is SO IMPORTANT. It can be lonely
finding those friends, but never give up and when you've found
them, love them up. Check in on the job interview, ask if their
kids are feeling better and write and just say hi. Both of you will
get joy from it and, boy, isn't the world a better place when it's
full of happy people.'—Stace

And finally . . . have more fun!

I cannot think of a better way to finish a book about balance, the
mental load and offloading the stress of it all than to talk about
fun . . . with a capital F. Seriously, where has all the fun gone in
our lives? When was the last time you made time to have fun?
Combine fun with a friend, and it's a double whammy hit for
your wellbeing.

What does fun look like in your life? Real fun. Joy. Laughter.
That moment when you're completely in your 'flow', when mira-
culously the mental load is lost and you're focusing on the pure
joy of the present moment. In their book *The Power Of Moments*,
the Heath brothers, Chip and Dan, have a sweet term called
'breaking the script', which they use to describe 'experiences that
rise above the routine. They make us feel engaged, joyful, amazed,
motivated.' Parties, road trips, weddings, spontaneous barbecues
and the like—it's about recognising your own script, and playing
with, poking and disrupting it. 'Not all the time—just enough to
keep those brown shoes looking fresh,' they write. 'By breaking
the script we can lay down a richer set of memories.'

You get comfortable when things are locked in, but how
alive do you feel when they are spontaneous? I had one of these

moments while writing this book. A friend of mine, Kel, who I've known since I was sixteen when we chopped salads in a healthy takeaway shop on weekends, randomly invited Tom and I on a boat to celebrate her birthday. I see her perhaps once or twice a year, so we're not familiar with many of her friends. As the night unfolded and, yes, hello champagne, we danced on the deck for hours, and I thought, *This is what life used to be like. FUN.* I felt human. I felt like *me* again—not someone's mum, someone's deadline. Sure, I was having a flood of feel-good chemicals from the company (and, yes, booze) but seriously, without the help of booze your brain releases those neurotransmitters anyway when you're letting loose.

It reminded me how seldom I do this, and how vital it is to have fun—to break your script—whatever that looks like for you. Making time for fun is a must-do. It's easy to let go of the things we love to do (the stuff that fills your cup) when we're overwhelmed, stressed, anxious and unbalanced. That wondrous feeling of losing ourselves in good quality fun reminds us that, despite all the B.S. that life throws at us, we can hold it together today, tomorrow and beyond. We can and will carry on.

'I personally don't think balance is bullshit but I have close friends who think it is . . . I have created a life so I can bring 100 per cent to each of those things that I love. Balance is beautiful, as long as we create it for ourselves and not for what other people think it should be. That's where we fall down. Someone else's balance is bullshit.'

Kemi Nekvapil, executive and personal coach

CHAPTER FOURTEEN

THIS WILL HAVE TO DO

So, here we are at that small chapter at the end where you share all your own learnings. (I just didn't want to use that dreary old word, 'epilogue'.)

My sister-in-law, Ness, and I had a fierce conversation (with wine on the couch) as I was finishing the manuscript for this book. She's a strong feminist at heart and I love her for that. She was worried that my focus on our health and wellbeing in Part Two might seem as if I was advocating for women to let go of the feminist fight. To accept that we're going to be overwhelmed and learn a few tricks to help deal with it. I reminded her that there is no miracle cure-all, that in order to keep up the fight we need help *now*. That even small steps towards true wellbeing are invaluable. She reiterated that we cannot just step away from our rage; we still need to fly our flags high and proud. She's absolutely right . . . not only do we need to talk (hello, Part One), we need to keep talking.

I want this book to inspire women, you, to start talking about these issues. Have the fierce conversations you need to have, with the people you need to have them with: partners, colleagues, bosses, kids, friends—so change starts to happen and momentum builds. But don't lose sight of this: right now, today, at this moment . . . some things have to give. Or your mental wellbeing suffers.

Writing this book has been one of the hardest things I've done in my twenty-year career—I had to be vulnerable, work hard on being a good-enough-ist, let go of my perfectionism and focus on processing the ideas and thoughts for discussion (my brain hurt sometimes). The conversation is ongoing: you'll never be able to tick the 'balanced' box as done—but you might find pockets of balance; moments of clarity amid the chaos. There is no perfect solution to this overwhelm we find ourselves in. There are no easy answers. No one's overwhelm is the same. So, people, this will have to do . . .

LET'S RALLY EACH OTHER

It's a bit messy right now—feminism. We have women *and* men who fly the pink flag, but we all struggle with the reality of it, daily. We probably knew it would be like this; it takes generations to figure out and shift deep cultural norms. But here's a fact that we can't ignore: women's wellbeing is declining and living in a constant state of overwhelm is making us sick. Women (and some men) are facing unprecedented pressures as they juggle work, children, their own relationships, ageing parents and other societal demands. The treadmill is gaining speed and in some cases we're flying off. We're over the overwhelm, fed up with the mental load sucking the life out of us. So, here's what we need to do: rally. No more blaming, just rally. Rally the men in our lives—husbands, brothers, dads, workmates and beyond—this is where the gender equality conversations need to ramp up, where men need to step up. We don't want a fight, we don't need any more fractured relationships. We need to empower men to be feminist role models for their kids. Some blokes are leading the charge; others need timely reminders that gender equality is, in fact, better for them.

We can do this together . . . not just for our own mental wellbeing but for our daughters, daughters-in-law, sons and the women, and men, of the future.

LET'S CARRY EACH OTHER

Women have been balancing work and life for yonks, but today our tribes are shrinking—our friends busier, our neighbours nameless and our families often scattered across different states or countries, too far away to help. The expectations on us are higher, we are leaning in, plugged in and chipping in more than ever before. So, what gives? Sadly, our friends. When we're lost in the trenches of unpaid work, when we are over capacity, the one thing we need more than ever is face-to-face connection, which is too often the first thing to go. Step away from the mindless scrolling, the quick texts and make the call. Pick up the phone and just say, 'Hi, how are you?' Healthy relationships are like therapy for your soul. As we carry on, we need to carry each other. And fun, let's not forget to have glorious, stupendous, ridiculous fun.

HAVE *YOUR* ALL

Gloria Steinem said it best: 'You can't do it all. No one can have two full-time jobs, have perfect children and cook three meals and be multi-orgasmic 'til dawn . . . Superwoman is the adversary of the women's movement.'

Let's work on ditching this tag from our vocab and social media and stop wearing those cute slogan T-shirts. It's making too many of us feel like crap. You simply can't be everything and do everything for everyone—boundaries, people, boundaries. Get comfortable saying no. You are good enough just as you are, doing your best in that moment (remember, bring on your A game—I'm winking at you right now). Use your values to pick your version of 'having it all'. This, in turn, means you will take on less. Our kids don't need to be in a million sports. One is good. We don't need to build a multi-million-dollar company. A flourishing smaller one is just as good. We don't need to make fancy, healthy meals every night. One a week is good. It's okay to not do it all; in fact, often we're happier when we do less.

DEFINE WELLNESS, FOR YOU

The antidote to overwhelm is finding your own meaning of wellness. True wellness is not what an Instagram-type spruiks or about putting on the right wellness-wear or using some herbal nose squirty thing—no, that's a twisted, commercialised idea. Although, I will buy into that sometimes because it just makes me feel . . . nice. True wellness is about getting the basic bits right—the mental, physical, spiritual and emotional—then the wellbeing bit will follow. It's also about living life wholeheartedly. That's how I see it. Oh, and don't be sold 'wellness' as a cure-all product—value good health instead.

TAKE MENTAL SPACE FROM YOUR MENTAL LOAD

When I was writing the final bit of this book, I had a few days by myself in Sydney while Tom and the kids stayed in his hometown of Adelaide. I unplugged my phone, disconnected with the outside world and bashed out the last few chapters of this book. Sure, I was working but I also had the gift of mental space. En route to the airport to pick them all up, I had this weird ah-ha moment where I noted: 'So, I am getting ready to go pick them all up and I find myself automatically switching on my mental load as the hours tick closer. It is a WEIRD feeling now that I am very AWARE of it.

But I find it hard to stop myself. I have not thought about anything but myself for the past five days, but now I am starting to think, okay, I need to pack for going away, I need to make sure Tom gets a present for his brother (like, he can think about that but I still do it!), what will we buy for dinner tonight before the shops shut, when will I do the washing from Adelaide . . . it is almost a surreal out-of-mind experience I am having. But, I am now AWARE, and I have to compartmentalise that in a part of my brain as I still want to finish my book with clear thinking.'

Mental space can be a moment, a minute or much longer than a week . . . but we all need it to move forward with clarity.

GRATITUDE CHANGES EVERYTHING

Gratitude is the most powerful tool there is when we actually *feel* it.

BALANCE LIVES IN THE PRESENT MOMENT

Balance is a state of consciousness that you choose. When you're caught in a hurricane, a storm or daily tremors, don't panic. See the balance in the moment, hold on tight to the sweet spot. Life will ebb and flow—there will be moments of madness, sadness and calm. It's about harnessing the calm when you're in it, and reminding yourself of that feeling when you're mentally overloaded. Overwhelm is a state of consciousness, and being conscious can help get you out.

DONE IS BETTER THAN PERFECT

Many brilliant writers and leaders have used these words in an assortment of ways. 'Done is better than good' (Elizabeth Gilbert), 'Done is better than perfect' (Jamila Rizvi and Sheryl Sandberg),

'Near enough is good enough' (Magda Szubanski). Hang onto this mantra as you bumble along in your life. This does not mean doing a mediocre job or producing a poor-quality product. Being done and finishing a task gives you an outcome. The result will give you insight into whether you've won (yes) or failed (also, yes) and from here you can decide on your next step.

So, that's it. It's time to say goodbye. And thank you for reading. I hope the words in this book, the wisdom and advice, have helped inspire you—to bring you more clarity, courage, confidence and determination to inspire more connection. Remember, you have the internal resources and you know your own experiences; your relationships that truly matter. You know what it takes to be a good enough human, mum, partner, work colleague, friend and so on. You know how to say no. Because at the end of the day, we all want to look up at the blue sky more often, wine in one hand, our other arm around our loved ones, and say, this is my life—no B.S.—and I *love* it.

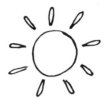

'Life is amazing. And then it's awful. And then it's amazing again. And in between the amazing and awful it's ordinary and mundane and routine. Breathe in the amazing, hold on through the awful, and relax and exhale during the ordinary. That's just living heartbreaking, soul-healing, amazing, awful, ordinary life. And it's breathtakingly beautiful.'

L.R. Knost, author and social justice advocate

IF YOU NEED SOME HELP

LIFELINE

Best for 24-hour crisis support: 13 11 14

lifeline.org.au

BEYOND BLUE

Whatever your age or stage, these guys can help you achieve your best mental health.

beyondblue.org.au

BLACK DOG INSTITUTE

It's worth noting they have an online anxiety self-test.

blackdoginstitute.org.au

MUMSPACE

This one is for the new parents among us.

mumspace.com.au

YOUR FRIENDS

Remember, being vulnerable with your friends isn't easy but let them in a tiny bit and it might just be the wellbeing boost you need.

NOTES OF GRATITUDE

To my kids, Jimmy, Hugo and Arabella, who might be cursing the end of this book as it means less iPad time and more mum time. 'How many words to go now, Mum?' became the question of the day during the months I spent on this book. 'Er, only 65,489 to go,' was my first reply. The last: '101!'

To Mum and Dad (Sheena and Kevin), who taught me the true meaning of life: family. Thank you for your unwavering support, unconditional love, steadfast values . . . and for being my best role models in life.

To Ange, Bo and Lizie—love you to bits, siblings, you awesome humans. All three of you forever inspire me.

Big thanks to Carly, who ran our household and watched the kids while I squirrelled away hours in the library. She is an integral part of my village.

To my besties, Rach, Chloe and Dana, thank you for the constant stream of 'checking in' texts. You always have my back (and I, yours).

To Tara, Ash and Stace. You guys rock.

To the inspiring celebrities, leaders and experts in their field. Thank you for your time, insights and wisdom. I'm forever inspired by you all.

To the *whimn* team who put up with me being AWOL while writing this book—thanks. I'm back . . .

Thank you to Andrea McNamara, officially my publishing consultant and editor. Unofficially a rock-solid steerer of the ship, a cheerleader, confidence hustler, all-round wise woman and a caring soul who is truly empathetic to the modern-day juggle. Thanks for sticking by me.

And Inga Berthold, thank you for your delightful illustrations. I love them.

Thanks to Kelly Fagan at Allen & Unwin for believing in this book, and giving me the opportunity to practise what I preach. Tessa Feggans for her kindness and understanding that my juggle is real and Isabelle O'Brien for her PR magic.

Finally—and most importantly—to my husband, Tom. My rock and feminist ally. My inspiration. My soulmate. Thank you for stepping up and carrying the load when I needed it most. I couldn't do this thing called life without you by my side.

ABOUT THE EXPERTS

Dr Marian Baird

Marian is a Professor of Gender and Employment Relations at the University of Sydney – the first female professor in industrial relations at the uni. She is one of Australia's leading researchers in the area of women, work and care and has won a slew of awards (including an AO) for improving the quality of women's working lives. In 2018 she was named one of the world's most influential people in gender equality policy by Apolitical, a London-based network that assists public servants to resolve major social challenges. She has four kids. Hear more from Marian on Twitter @ProfMarianBaird.

Lola Berry

Lola is a leading Australian nutritionist, author, yoga teacher and former owner of smoothie bar, Happy Place. Her latest business venture is Lola Coffee. She appears regularly on *Studio 10, The Project*, *The Today Show* and *A Current Affair*. She has penned eleven books and hosts a podcast called *Fearlessly Failing*. She is a qualified vinyasa and yin yoga teacher. Hear more from Lola on Instagram @yummololaberry.

Jane Caro

Jane is a pro at spinning professional plates: author of nine books (including my favourite *Accidental Feminists*), novelist, MC, lecturer, mentor, TV social commentator, columnist, workshop facilitator, speaker, broadcaster and award-winning advertising writer and Walkley Award recipient. Phew. In 2019, she was appointed a Member of the Order of Australia (AM) for her service to the broadcast media. She also revels in grandmother duties. Hear more from Jane on Twitter @JaneCaro.

Alison Hill

Ali is the CEO of Pragmatic Thinking, a three-times listed *Australian Financial Review* Fast 100 company. She's a psycho-logist, award-winning businesswoman, speaker and producer and host of *Stand Out Life* podcast. She is a regular on the media circuit, a bestselling author and a world-class dancer in her own kitchen (much to the embarrassment of her two kids). Find out more: alisonhill.com.au.

Dr Rebecca Huntley

Rebecca is a leading social researcher and expert on Australia's social trends with degrees in law, a first-class degree in film studies and a PhD in gender studies. She is the author of numerous books, including her 2019 Quarterly Essay, *Australia Fair: Listening to the nation*. She is a presenter for ABC's Radio National. She is a marriage celebrant and mum to three girls. Hear more from Rebecca on Twitter @RebeccaHuntley2.

Dana Kerford

Dana is a teacher, friendship expert and founder of URSTRONG, a global social-emotional wellbeing program for kids. She is a regular media spokeswoman and presenter at education conferences around the world. She has two kids, lives in Noosa and loves drinking wine with friends. Find out more: urstrong.com.

Ginni Mansberg

Ginni is a practising GP and regular TV doctor (*Embarrassing Bodies Down Under*, *Sunrise*, *The Morning Show* and *Things You Can't Talk About On TV*). The Sydneysider is a medical journalist and columnist and the author of *The M Word: How to Thrive in Menopause* (2019). She is co-founder of Evidence Skin Care (ESK). She juggles life with all her kids, is a wannabe Masterchef and dedicated caffeine addict. Hear more from Dr Ginni on Twitter @Dr_Ginni.

Emma Murray

Emma is a psychotherapist, mindfulness coach, NLP master practitioner and clinical hypnotherapist who has been working with elite athletes, corporate executives and students for more than twenty years. She was considered the 'secret weapon' behind Richmond Football Club's drought-breaking AFL premiership in 2017. The former national-level netball player has four kids and lives in Melbourne. Hear more from Emma on Instagram @em.murray.1.

Kemi Nekvapil

Kemi is an executive and personal coach and 'Dare to Lead' facilitator who has worked in the wellness industry for more than twenty years. She is an ICF-accredited life coach, speaker and regular media commentator. She has penned two books, *Raw Beauty* and *The Gift Of Asking,* and has a podcast, *The Shift Series.* When not working, the mum of two gets lost in her garden. Find out more: keminekvapil.com.

Leah Ruppanner

Leah is an Associate Professor of Sociology and Co-Director of The Policy Lab at the University of Melbourne. She's an expert in family, gender, public policy, cross-national research and quantitative methods. She writes regularly for *The Conversation* and her book, *Boxed Out: Barriers to mothers' employment across U.S. states*, will be published by Temple University Press in 2020. She has a sweet side hustle—she owns a brewery in South Melbourne. Hear more from Leah on Twitter @leahruppanner.

Libby Weaver

Libby is one of Australia's leading nutritional biochemists. She's a speaker, founder of the plant-based supplement range, Bio Blends, and author of thirteen books which have sold more than 450,000 copies across New Zealand and Australia. In fact, Hugh Jackman and Deborra-Lee Furness describe her as a 'one stop shop in achieving and maintaining ultimate health and wellbeing'. Hear more from Dr Libby on Instagram @drlibby.

ENDNOTES

A BIT ABOUT THIS BOOK

p. xi   rate of depression and anxiety in Australian women: Australian Bureau of Statistics, *National Health Survey: First Results—Australia 2017–18* (NHS 2017–18), Canberra

1: HONESTLY, IS THIS WHAT WE WERE PROMISED?

p. 9   'thought there was something wrong with me . . .': Betty Friedan, on writing *The Feminine Mystique*, 'Up from the kitchen floor', *The New York Times*, 4 March 1973

p. 10   'Since marriage constitutes slavery for women . . .': Sheila Cronin, in 'Marriage', essay, 1970

p. 10   'Friedan was concerned . . .': Brigid Schulte, *Overwhelmed,* Picador, USA, 2015, p. 121

p. 11   'nicely nicely, softly softly': 'Clementine Ford: "There's something really toxic with the way men bond in Australia"', *The Guardian Australia*, 28 September 2016

p. 12   'Because the purpose of feminism . . .': Caitlin Moran, *How To Be A Woman,* Ebury Press, 2011, p. 88

p. 12   'Sure, the gender pay gap is still at 14 per cent . . .': Workplace Gender Equality Agency, gender pay gap statistics, 15 August 2019

p. 12   'And yes, it is having children . . .': 'Children and gender inequality: evidence from Denmark', published by the US National Bureau of Economic Research, 2018

2: THE PARADOX OF HAVING IT ALL, BUT STILL WANTING MORE

p. 16   'Marriage still ain't equal . . .': Michelle Obama, quoted in 'Michelle Obama got especially comfortable during her book-tour stop in Brooklyn', *Vanity Fair*, 2 December 2018

p. 19   'More choices may not always mean more control': Barry Schwartz, *The Paradox of Choice: Why More Is Less,* Harper Perennial, 2004, p. 108

p. 20   'women's happiness has declined . . .': Betsey Stevenson and Justin Wolfers, 'The paradox of declining female happiness', *American Economic Journal: Economic Policy*, Volume 1, Issue 2, 2009, pp. 190–225.

p. 21 'women are paying an even higher price than men . . .': Arianna Huffington, 'The Third Women's Revolution', Thrive Global, 9 March 2017

p. 22 'health and wellbeing of young women . . .': *Growing up unequal,* issues paper by Women's Health Victoria, April 2018

p. 22 'Many of these women are worrying not about having it all . . .': Anne-Marie Slaughter, 'Why women still can't have it all', *The Atlantic,* July/August 2012

p. 24 'a state of wellbeing . . .': World Health Organization (WHO), <who.int/mental_health/who_urges_investment/en/>

p. 24 'nearly one in two females . . .': figures from 2007 National Survey of Mental Health and Wellbeing and the NHS 2017–18, quoted in web report 'The health of Australia's females', Australian Institute of Health And Welfare, <aihw.gov.au/reports/men-women/female-health/contents/who-are>

p. 24 'mood disorders continue to be more common amongst women than men': ABS, *Australian Health Survey: First Results,* Black Dog Institute, Canberra, 2012

p. 25 'critical determinant of mental health and mental illness': World Health Organization (WHO), <who.int/mental_health/prevention/genderwomen/en/>

p. 25 'more women (14.5 per cent) than men . . .': ABS, *National Health Survey: First Results—Australia 2017–18,* Canberra, quoted by Beyond Blue, <www.beyondblue.org.au/media/statistics>

p. 25 'one in five mothers of children aged 24 months . . .': perinatal depression data from the 2010 Australian National Infant Feeding Survey, Australian Institute of Health and Welfare, 2012, quoted by Black Dog Institute

p. 26 one of the biggest national health studies: Women's Health Survey 2018, Jean Hailes for Women's Health, <jeanhailes.org.au/contents/documents/News/Womens-Health-Survey-Report-web.pdf>

p. 30 'Almost every woman I have seen in my office . . .': Louann Brizendine, *The Female Brain,* Broadway Books, 2006, p. 210

3: THE I'M-TOO-BLOODY-EXHAUSTED GENERATION

p. 36 'a human received . . .': Martin Hilbert, 'The world's technological capacity to store, communicate, and compute information', *Science,* 1 April 2011

p. 37 'In order to understand one person . . .': Daniel J. Levitin, *The Organized Mind,* Dutton Penguin Random House, 2014, <penguin.com/ajax/books/excerpt/9780147516312>

p. 37 we check our phones every twelve minutes: from a 2017 US study by global tech protection and support company Asurion, <nypost.com/2017/11/08/americans-check-their-phones-80-times-a-day-study/>

p. 41 'Technology spins that overwhelm faster': Brigid Schulte, *Overwhelmed,* Picador USA, 2015 p. 26

p. 43   'Technology has changed our expectations . . .': Sally-Anne Blanshard in 'Why hustle culture is making me feel pretty crappy', *whimn*, 22 May 2019

p. 44   'in our culture, "mom" has been deemed . . .': Eve Rodsky, *Fair Play*, Penguin Random House, 2019, p. 31

p. 44   'Eight hours of paid employment . . .': from a University of Cambridge study, *Social Science and Medicine*, 18 June 2019, <sciencedaily.com/ releases/2019/06/190618192030.htm>

p. 45   'It sounds like the answer to balance . . .': Andrea Cross, quoted by Wendy Tuohy and Kasey Edwards, 'The four-day fallacy: busting the myth of part-time working mums', *Sydney Morning Herald*, 8 September 2019

p. 47   'a syndrome conceptualised as . . .': WHO, 11th Revision of the *International Classification of Diseases* (ICD-11), QD85 Burn-out, May 2019

p. 48   'one of the most widely discussed . . .': Linda and Torsten Heinemann, 'Burnout research: Emergence and scientific investigation of a contested diagnosis', *SAGE Open*, SAGE Journals, January–March 2017

p. 48   'women suffer from alarmingly higher rates of burnout . . .': Beauregard et al., 'Gendered pathways to burnout', results from the SALVEO Study, 2018, <ncbi.nlm.nih.gov/pubmed/29471461>

4: THE SECOND SHIFT

p. 53   'The average Australian father . . .': Annabel Crabb, *Men At Work: Australia's Parenthood Trap,* Quarterly Essay QE75, Black Inc., September 2019, p. 35

p. 53   'The day-in, day-out work of parenting . . .': Jane Caro, *Accidental Feminists*, Melbourne University Publishing, 2019, p. 78

p. 56   'Work that produces goods or services . . .': OECD, Glossary of statistical terms, updated 2013, <stats.oecd.org/glossary/>

p. 56   women spend more time doing unpaid . . . : 2016 Australian Census, ABS and *Household, Income and Labour Dynamics in Australia Survey*, aka the HILDA Survey, <melbourneinstitute.unimelb.edu.au/hilda>

p. 59   mothers are 18 per cent more stressed: statistics from the UK Household Longitudinal Survey, the largest survey of its kind in the world

p. 59   'Women have to find ways to combine housework . . .': Dr Inga Lass, quoted by Natalic Rcilly, 'The increased stress felt by working mothers has finally been measured', *Sydney Morning Herald*, 6 February 2019

p. 59   'shit I do' list: Eve Rodsky, *Fair Play*, Penguin Random House, 2019, p. 34

p. 61   two-thirds of the 6289 working parents surveyed: *National Working Families Report 2019*, research from the inaugural National Working Families Survey conducted by Parents At Work, <parentsandcarersatwork.com/wp-content/ uploads/2019/10/NWFSurvey-Executive-Summary.pdf>

5: THE PROBLEM THAT NOW HAS A NAME

p. 70   'We lend an ear . . .': Gemma Hartley, *Fed Up: Emotional Labor, Women and the Way Forward*, HarperOne, 2018, p. 11

p. 70   'When you live by yourself . . .': Abbey Lenton, 'We need to talk about the mental load of living solo', *whimn*, 18 October 2019

p. 71   the concept of 'emotional labour': Arlie Russell Hochschild, *The Managed Heart*, Berkeley: The University of California Press, 1983

p. 71   women do, in fact, carry more of the mental load: Susan Walzer, 'Thinking About The Baby: Gender and divisions of infant care', *Social Problems*, Volume 43, Issue 2, 1 May 1996, pp. 219–34

p. 71   men's 'privileged status': Marci D. Cottingham, Rebecca J. Erickson and James M. Diefendorff, 'Examining men's status shield and status bonus', *Sex Roles*, Volume 72, Issues 7–8, 2015, pp. 377–89

p. 71   'The mental load means . . .': Emma, 'You Should've Asked':

p. 72   'one of the most important gender-equity issues . . .': Darcy Lockman, 'What "good" dads get away with', *The New York Times*, 4 May 2019

p. 74   'gender stereotyping is rife in advertising': *Community Responses to Gender Portrayals in Advertising*, RMIT and Women's Health Victoria (WHV), October 2019

p. 74   'In an era where "good" mothers are those . . .': Leah Ruppanner for podcast *Ladies, We Need To Talk*, ABC Radio, 14 September 2017

p. 78   'In general, when people spend a lot of time . . .': David Ginsberg, Director of Research, and Moira Burke, Research Scientist, Facebook, blog post, 15 December 2017

p. 79   social media can still have a negative effect . . . : Hui-Tzu Chou and Nicholas Edge, '"They are happier and having better lives than I am": The impact of using Facebook on perceptions of others' lives', *Cyberpsychology, Behavior, and Social Networking*, Volume 15, No. 2, 2012, pp. 117–21

6: #SUPERWOMAN, WE HAVE A PROBLEM

p. 85   the cult of intensive motherhood: Brigid Schulte, *Overwhelmed*, Picador USA, 2015, p. 179

p. 85   so-called impostor syndrome: P. R. Clance and S. A. Imes, 'The Impostor Phenomenon In High Achieving Women: Dynamics and therapeutic intervention', *Psychotherapy: Theory, Research & Practice*, Volume 15, Issue 3, 1978, pp. 241–47

p. 86   'How very many layers we operate on . . .': Elizabeth Gilbert, *Eat, Pray, Love*, Bloomsbury, 2007, p. 51

p. 88 high social expectations on young women: Dr Blashki, quoted by Kate Aubusson, 'It's not easy being a young woman these days', *Sydney Morning Herald*, 23 October 2019

p. 88 'As a woman, making an effort isn't good enough . . .': Gemma Hartley, *Fed Up: Emotional Labor, Women and the Way Forward*, HarperOne, 2018, p. 87

p. 90 a study of 4000 Americans: Hal E. Hershfield, Cassie Mogilner and Uri Barnea, 'People who choose time over money are happier', SAGE Journals, Volume 7, Issue: 7, 25 May 2016, pp. 697–706

p. 91 parents spend twice as much time with their children: *The Economist*, 27 November 2017

p. 92 time is the perfect equaliser: Marilyn Waring, discussed by Anne Manne in 'Making women's unpaid work count', *The Monthly*, May 2018

p. 94 Dr Ginni Mansberg, *The M Word: How to Thrive in Menopause*, Murdoch Books, 2020

p. 95 women consistently report higher stress levels: research reported in *Journal of Brain and Behavior*, 5 June 2016, <doi.org/10.1002/brb3.497>

7: THE WELLNESS SOLUTION

p. 103 'exciting field of wellness enhancement': Robert Rodale, quoted by Ben Zimmer, *The New York Times Magazine*, 16 April 2010

p. 104 'The minute the phrase "having it all" lost favor . . .': Taffy Brodesser-Akner, 'How Goop's haters made Gwyneth Paltrow's company worth $250 million', *The New York Times Magazine*, 25 July 2018

p. 106 'the wellness industry is now worth US$4.5 trillion . . .': <globalwellnessinstitute.org/industry-research/>

p. 108 'Every field of knowledge requires . . .': Dr Karl Kruszelnicki, *Vital Science*, Pan Macmillan, 2018, p. 79

p. 109 'feminist wellness' as one of the top ten global trends: 2018 *Global Wellness Trends Report* drawn from the Global Wellness Summit and professionals in the wellness industry

p. 112 Australia has one of the highest life expectancies: World Health Rankings, 2018 <worldlifeexpectancy.com/australia-life-expectancy>

p. 112 two thirds of Australian adults are overweight: ABS, *National Health Survey: First Results—Australia 2017–18*, 4364.0.55.001

p. 113 the tribe who 'gets' the health and wellness lifestyle: Women's Health Survey 2018, Jean Hailes for Women's Health, p.4, <jeanhailes.org.au/contents/documents/News/Womens-Health-Survey-Report-web.pdf>

8: THE B.S. OF IT ALL

p. 122 health is the new black: research conducted by the research department at Pacific Magazines, Sydney, around 2014–16

p. 123 'I called this poisonous relationship . . .': Jessica Knoll, 'Smash The Wellness Industry', *The New York Times*, 8 June 2019

p. 125 'Health is now advertised as a project . . .': Dr Nikki Stamp, *Pretty Unhealthy: Why our obsession with looking healthy is making us sick*, Murdoch Books, 2019

p. 126 'And there is a gendered claw . . .': Eva Wiseman, 'Is this the end of wellness?', *The Guardian*, 14 July 2019

p. 126 Dopamine, balance for wellbeing: '10 Best Ways to Increase Dopamine Levels Naturally', *healthline.com*, May 2018, based on data supplied by US National Library of Medicine, National Institutes of Health

p. 131 'healthy work–life integration': Arianna Huffington, 'How millennials can create healthy work–life integration', 'Wisdom' post on *Thrive Global*, 10 May 2017

p. 131 'It's when you have so much to do . . .': Sarah Wilson, *First, We Make The Beast Beautiful*, Pan Macmillan, 2017, p. 232

p. 133 'Wellbeing means people living lives of purpose . . .': quoted by Eleanor Ainge Roy in 'New Zealand's world-first "wellbeing" budget to focus on poverty and mental health', *The Guardian Australia*, 14 May 2019

9: CLARITY: THE COUNTERBALANCE

p. 141 Mark Manson, *The Subtle Art of Not Giving a Fuck: A counterintuitive approach to living a good life*, HarperOne, 2016

p. 142 'What I know for sure is that speaking your truth is the most powerful tool we all have': Oprah Winfrey, <youtube.com/watch?v=z84UtPAWqNM>

p. 144 'The alternative [to having it all] . . .': Sandra Sdraulig, quoted by Annie Brown, 'There's no "right" time to have a baby, just ask the "millennial Oprah"', *Sydney Morning Herald*, 24 September 2019

p. 147 'When you're burnt out . . .': Emilie Aries, 'The biggest falsehood about burnout', *Bossed Up*, Ingram Publisher Services US, 31 January 2019, <bossedup.org/episode93/>

p. 152 the value of the meditation market globally: 'The U.S. Meditation Market' report, Marketdata Enterprises, Inc., September 2017, <webwire.com/ViewPressRel.asp?aId=214152>

p. 152 'the average brain generates . . .': Jane Martino and James Tutton, *Smiling Mind: mindfulness made easy*, Hardie Grant Books, 2015, p. 22

10: THE UNDENIABLE THRILL OF CREATING MENTAL SPACE

p. 164 Creating a mental or physical anchor . . . : <blog.smilingmind.com.au/how-to-mindful-parenting>

p. 164 mindfulness meditation as a cure: Alvin Powell, 'When science meets mindfulness', *The Harvard Gazette*, 9 April 2018

p. 168 'The point here is to challenge your assumptions . . .': Marie Forleo, <marieforleo.com/2011/02/deal-overwhelm-free-video-workshop/>

p. 170 'Personal autonomy is what makes us . . .': Nelly Thomas, 'The benefits of taking mum vacations by yourself', *ABC Life*, 30 September 2019

p. 172 exercise is a scientifically backed mood booster: 'Working Out Boosts Brain Health', Rod K. Dishman and Mark Sothmann, published online by the American Psychological Association, 4 March 2020, <apa.org/helpcenter/exercise-stress>

p. 173 'Green exercise': 'The mental and physical health outcomes of green exercise', first published on PubMed.gov, The National Center for Biotechnology Information, October 2005, <ncbi.nlm.nih.gov/pubmed/16416750>

11: WHEN COURAGE CAN CURE

p. 184 'Perfectionism is a self-destructive . . .': Brené Brown, *Daring Greatly*, Penguin, 2012, p. 130

p. 184 'For women, shame is . . .': Brené Brown, *The Gifts of Imperfection*, Hazelden Publishing, 2010

p. 185 'The things you think you wouldn't be able to survive . . .': Leigh Sales, *Any Ordinary Day*, Penguin Random House, 2019, p. 238

p. 185 comprehensive study of life satisfaction: David G. Blanchflower and Andrew Oswald, 'Is well-being U-shaped over the life cycle?', *National Bureau of Economic Research*, NBER Working Paper No. 12935, February 2007

p. 187 'I have always been . . .': 'How I learnt to break up with "perfection sickness"', *Body+Soul*, whimn, 21 August 2019

p. 188 'It's also why the most common answer . . .': Gemma Hartley, *Fed Up: Emotional Labor, Women and the Way Forward*, HarperOne, 2018, p. 72

p. 189 'Trying to do it all . . .': Sheryl Sandberg, *Lean In*, Knopf, 2013

p. 190 'In order to set boundaries that stick . . .': Alison Hill, *Stand Out*, John Wiley & Sons Australia, 2016, p. 48

p. 198 overcoming the negative bias: Martin Seligman, *Learned Optimism,* Alfred A. Knopf, 1991

p. 199 'gratitude helps people feel more positive emotions . . .': 'In Praise of Gratitude', Harvard Health Publishing, Harvard Medical School, 5 June 2019

p. 199 'Gratitude is long lasting . . .': Janice Kaplan, *The Gratitude Diaries: How a year looking on the bright side transformed my life,* Dutton, 2015, p. 14

12: OWN YOUR CONFIDENCE

p. 204 'I very much believe . . .': Zoë Foster Blake, quoted by Bridie Jabour, 'Zoë Foster Blake on "chronic over-busyness": "I wish I could just stop sometimes"', *The Guardian Australia*, 15 February 2019

p. 206 'I think the most stressful thing . . .': Beyoncé, quoted in 'Ask Me Anything', *Elle*, 9 December 2019, <elle.com/culture/celebrities/a29999871/beyonce-ivy-park-adidas-interview/>

p. 207 only 20 per cent of Australian women have high self-esteem: *Dove Global Beauty and Confidence Report,* Dove Global Beauty, 21 June 2016, <prnewswire.com/in/news-releases/new-dove-research-finds-beauty-pressures-up-and-women-and-girls-calling-for-change-583743771>

p. 208 'Confidence is the stuff . . .': Katty Kay and Claire Shipman, *The Confidence Code,* HarperCollins, 2014, p. 50

p. 208 putting confidence in your spotlight: adapted from Harriet Griffey, *I Want To Be Confident: Living, working and communicating with confidence,* Hardie Grant, 2017

p. 210 'Beware of the insidious power . . .': Jennifer S. Mills and others, '"Selfie" harm: Effects on mood and body image in young women', *ScienceDirect*, 24 August 2018, <sciencedirect.com/science/article/pii/S1740144517305326>

p. 211 'We found that cueing people to reflect . . .': research referenced by Ozlem Ayduk and Ethan Kross, 'Pronouns matter when psyching yourself up', *Harvard Business Review*, 6 February 2015

p. 213 'The source of self-sabotage . . .': Judy Ho, 'Why We Self-Sabotage', psychologytoday.com, 2 November 2019

p. 215 impostor syndrome at work: 'The high cost of perfectionism', Society for Industrial and Organizational Psychology, published at eurekalert.org, 12 July 2019

p. 215 'Confidence and leadership are muscles . . .': Sheryl Sandberg, quoted by Samantha Walravens in '5 Exercises Sheryl Sandberg, Silicon Valley Women Do to Build Confidence', forbes.com, 6 September 2016

p. 216 the confidence/competence loop: there are a lot of good online resources about making this loop work for you—google it

p. 217 Elizabeth Gilbert, *Big Magic: Creative Living Beyond Fear*, Bloomsbury, 2015

p. 218 'To stretch is to place ourselves in situations . . .': Chip Heath and Dan Heath, *The Power Of Moments*, Simon & Schuster, 2017, p. 117

p. 218 'In the process she learned more . . .': ibid, *The Power Of Moments*, p. 132

p. 219 'As women, we're encouraged to shrink . . .': Melissa Shedden, 'Why are women describing themselves as "appropriately confident"?', *whimn*, 30 October 2018

13: THE POWER OF CONNECTION

p. 230 'Most of us define the meaning of our lives . . .': Hugh Mackay, *What Makes Us Tick?,* Hachette, 2010, p. 113

p. 231 loneliness and link to health problems: a meta-analysis looking at 23 studies with more than 181,000 participants by N.K. Valtorta, M. Kanaan, S. Gilbody et al., 'Loneliness and social isolation as risk factors for coronary heart disease and stroke: systematic review and meta-analysis of longitudinal observational studies', *Heart*, Volume 102, Issue 13, 100916, 1 July 2016, <ncbi.nlm.nih.gov/pubmed/27091846>

p. 231 what keeps people happy and healthy: 'Good genes are nice, but joy is better', The Harvard Study of Adult Development, discussed by Liz Mineo, *The Harvard Gazette*, 11 April 2017

p. 231 'What Makes A Good Life?': TEDx Talk by Dr Robert Waldinger on lessons from the longest study on happiness, filmed November 2015, <ted.com/talks/robert_waldinger_what_makes_a_good_life_lessons_from_the_longest_study_on_happiness?language=en>

p. 232 'This back-and-forth is repeated . . .': Glennon Doyle, *Love Warrior*, Flatiron Books, 2016, p. 93

p. 234 'The greatest barriers to connection . . .': Hugh Mackay, *What Makes Us Tick?*, op cit, p. 115

p. 235 positivity, vulnerability and consistency in friendships: Shasta Nelson, *Frientimacy*, Seal Press, 2016

p. 237 'Abandon the cultural myth . . .': quoted in 'Roxane Gay: the bad feminist manifesto', *The Guardian*, 2 August 2014, an edited extract from Roxane Gay, *Bad Feminist*, Harper Perennial, 2014

p. 237 women supporting women: poll by Ellevate Network (leading network for professional women) and Berlin Cameron (creative agency), February 2019

p. 240 'breaking the script': Chip Heath and Dan Heath, *The Power Of Moments*, Simon & Schuster, 2017, p. 87